The Views and Experiences
of Disabled Children and Their Siblings

of related interest

Disabled Children and the Law
Research and Good Practice
Janet Read and Luke Clements
ISBN 1 85302 793 6

Choosing Assistive Devices
A Guide for Users and Professionals
Helen Pain, Lindsay McLellan and Sally Gore
ISBN 1 85302 985 8

Manual Handling in Health and Social Care
An A–Z of Law and Practice
Michael Mandelstam
ISBN 1 84310 041 X

Growing Up with Disability
Edited by Carol Robinson and Kirsten Stalker
ISBN 1 85302 568 2
Research Highlights in Social Work 34

Childhood Experiences of Domestic Violence
Caroline McGee
ISBN 1 85302 827 4

The Child's World
Assessing Children in Need
Edited by Jan Horwath
ISBN 1 85302 957 2

Reconceptualising Work with 'Carers'
New Directions for Policy and Practice
Edited by Kirsten Stalker
ISBN 1 84310 118 1
Research Highlights in Social Work 43

The Views and Experiences of Disabled Children and Their Siblings

A Positive Outlook

Clare Connors and Kirsten Stalker

Jessica Kingsley Publishers
London and Philadelphia

First published in the United Kingdom in 2003
by Jessica Kingsley Publishers Ltd
116 Pentonville Road
London N1 9JB, England
and
325 Chestnut Street
Philadelphia, PA 19106, USA
www.jkp.com

Copyright © 2003 Clare Connors and Kirsten Stalker

Library of Congress Cataloging in Publication Data

Conners, Clare, 1957-
  The experiences and views of disabled children and their siblings : implications for practice and policy / Clare Conners and Kirsten Stalker.
    p. cm.
  Includes bibliographical references and index.
  ISBN 1-84310-127-0 (pbk : alk. paper)
    1. Handicapped children--Attitudes. 2. Brothers and sisters--Attitudes. I. Stalker, Kirsten. II. Title.

HV888.C645 2002
362.4'083–dc21   2002038924

British Library Cataloguing in Publication Data
A CIP catalogue record for this book is available from the British Library

ISBN 1 84310 127 0

Printed and Bound in Great Britain by
Athenaeum Press, Gateshead, Tyne and Wear

Contents

List of Appendices

*This book is dedicated to the memory of
Maureen Oswin (1931–2001) who did so much
to make the lives of disabled children valued and ordinary.*

Acknowledgements

This study was carried out at the Social Work Research Centre at the University of Stirling as part of a research programme funded by the Central Research Unit of the Scottish Executive. We wish to thank the children and families who took part in the study for all their help and hospitality. We are especially grateful to Danielle Atai and Gemma Houldcroft who acted as advisers to the study and made very helpful suggestions about the research proposal and the materials. We are grateful to Enlighten for helping organise these meetings. Thanks also to Sheena Conroy, Cathy Murray, Rena Phillips, Samantha Punch, Caitlin Skinner and Nick Watson for their comments at an early stage. Particular thanks must go to Margaret Burt who conducted some of the interviews and to Lynne O'Rourke of Stirling University Media Services who was responsible for the graphic design of the materials. Last but not least, thanks to Pam Lavery and Sheena Conroy for secretarial support.

Glossary

The following glossary explains the words used throughout the text:

Disabled children
The study was broadly informed by the social model of disability. This points to constraints and barriers within society – material, social, cultural and attitudinal – as the cause of disability, rather than an individual's actual impairment. From this perspective, the term 'disabled children' is used in preference to 'children with disabilities'.

Complex support needs
This describes the needs some children had over and above their learning impairment. For example, some children also had physical and sensory impairments.

Inclusive setting
This refers to a mainstream school which includes disabled children.

Integrated setting
In this, children attend units attached to a mainstream school. Some children spend part of their day in mainstream.

Resourced school
A mainstream school which acts as a specialist setting for children with particular impairments. Some schools may be 'resourced' for children with physical impairments and some for sensory impairments.

Segregated setting
This is used to describe a special school.

Short-term breaks
Previously referred to as 'respite care' – a term which carries negative connotations, implying that parents need to have time off from the 'burden' of caring for their child.

Chapter One

The Policy and Research Background

Introduction

This book presents the findings from a two-year study, carried out from 1998 to 2000, exploring children's experiences of disability. The main aim was to examine disabled children's perceptions of the impact of disability on them. This is important because, although much has been written about parents' and professionals' views of the effects of disability on children, very few studies have sought children's views. Another aim was to explore the perceptions of children who have disabled brothers or sisters, to examine their views about the impact of having a disabled sibling. Again, this is important because most accounts of sibling experience and effect have been written from parental or professional viewpoints rather than by, or by asking, the brothers and sisters themselves. These questions are given added impetus by current childcare legislation in Britain which requires local authorities to 'minimise the effects of disability' on disabled children, and, in Scotland, on children 'adversely affected' by the disability of someone in their family. Yet little is known about these effects from the children's standpoint.

Twenty-six disabled children, aged between 7 and 15, and 24 of their brothers and sisters, aged from 5 to 19, were asked to talk about their day to day lives. The disabled children were asked about their likes and dislikes, their achievements, the barriers they faced, the support they received and

their future aspirations. Their siblings were asked about their relationships with the disabled child, the advantages and disadvantages, if any, of having a disabled sibling, what impact it had on them, and what information and support they received or wanted. Their parents were also interviewed, to seek their views about the children's experiences: they were not asked to talk about their own experiences of caring. The main focus throughout the study has been on the children's perspectives.

The aims of the study were as follows:

- to explore disabled children's understandings of disability

- to examine the ways in which they negotiate the experience of disability in their everyday lives

- to examine these children's perceptions of their relationships with professionals, and their knowledge and views of service provision

- to examine siblings' perceptions of the effects on them of having a disabled brother or sister

- to identify and draw out the implications for social work and health services, particularly in terms of minimising the effects on children of disability and enabling them to lead as 'ordinary' lives as possible, as set out in recent childcare legislation in the UK.

This chapter begins by reviewing recent policy developments which emphasise the importance of seeking the views of disabled children. It goes on to examine trends in the literature on families with disabled children, including the research on siblings, and some recent studies exploring the views of disabled children. Understandings of disability and childhood which guided this research are discussed. Chapter 2 describes how the study was carried out and the methods we used to communicate with the children.

The following chapters present the main findings of the research. Chapter 3 examines how disabled children negotiate day to day life at home while Chapter 4 looks at their experiences at school. Chapter 5 considers what the children had to say about services and professionals. Because many did not say a great deal on these subjects, in this chapter

more than others we draw on parents' accounts. Chapter 6 looks at the views and experiences of siblings. The next chapter explores the children's understandings and experiences of disability: this focuses on the disabled children but includes a section on siblings. The final chapter presents the main conclusions of the research and draws out implications for policy and practice.

The glossary at the beginning of the book explains certain key terms. To protect confidentiality, the real names of children, families and places have been changed, as have some minor biographical details. For the most part, children have been given more than one pseudonym to further protect their identity. There are a few exceptions, however, when we wanted the reader to follow an individual child, at least for part of the book, because of the significance of a particular point or feature of their circumstances.

The policy background

The development of support and services for disabled children has 'a history steeped in vacillating attitudes: extreme cruelty alternating with protection, neglect alternating with enlightened provision, exploitation alternating with respect' (Oswin 1998, p.29). Oswin traces that history from Ancient Greece to modern times. Her account shows how hostile and punitive practices have been interspersed with more benign approaches. For much of the 20th century, many parents were advised to place their disabled children in institutions from an early age: thus, thousands were brought up in 'colonies' or long-stay hospitals. Over the past 30 years or so, such institutions have gradually been closing down. The provision of full time education and a range of support services have enabled most parents to care for their children at home.

The late 20th century saw the rise of the consumer movement and a demand for civil rights on the part of minority groups. Article 12 of the United Nations Convention on the Rights of the Child (1989) states that children have the right to be consulted on any matter affecting them. Article 23 asserts that disabled children have the right to a full and decent life, to dignity and independence, and to be brought up in circumstances which enable their active participation in the community.

Historically, disabled children in Britain have been excluded from mainstream childcare legislation (Shearer 1980). Recent childcare law – the Children Act 1989, the Children (Scotland) Act 1995 and the Northern Ireland Children's Order 1995 – were important landmarks in that disabled children are fully included in their provisions. Disabled children are one of several groups classed as 'children in need' and as such are also affected by certain special provisions. The Acts embody several key principles in relation to disabled children, namely:

- promotion of their welfare
- normalisation/inclusion
- participation of the child
- partnership with parents
- interagency collaboration
- cultural sensitivity.

The Acts place a duty on local authorities to provide a range of services for children 'in need'. In England, Wales and Scotland, such services should be designed to minimise the effects on disabled children of their 'disabilities'; in Northern Ireland, there should be 'a range and level of services appropriate to these children's needs'. Local authorities are required to have 'due regard' for the views of the child in decisions affecting him or her. The Acts require authorities to publish children's services plans. In preparing these, authorities must consult children and their families who are using, have used or may be potential users of services.

Research into the implementation of the Children Act 1989 reported that some local authorities in England were not listening to disabled children. Both Morris (1998a) and the Social Services Inspectorate (1998) found little evidence that children's wishes and feelings about their placements were being ascertained. Morris spoke to 30 young people in residential homes and schools: they had experienced distress when separated from their families, when they were not consulted about short-term care arrangements, when their privacy was violated or they were treated disrespectfully by staff. Some social workers stated that certain children were too young or too disabled to voice an opinion. Little

effort had been made to find alternative ways of exploring their views. Other social workers did not think they had the necessary skills to work directly with children with communication difficulties. They lacked training in this area and it was not prioritised by managers (SSI 1998).

However, recent policy developments in the UK have shone a spotlight on children's services. In 1998, the Department of Health set up *Quality Protects*, a three-year initiative aimed at transforming services for children in need in England. Its objectives are to offer more effective protection, better quality care and improved life chances to disadvantaged and vulnerable children. Disabled children are a priority group and *Quality Protects* aims to ensure they 'gain maximum life chance benefits from educational opportunities, health care and social care, while living with their families or in other appropriate settings in the community where their assessed needs are adequately met and reviewed' (DoH 1998 p.1). These objectives are reiterated in the Government's strategy for people with learning disabilities. The White Paper (DoH 2001) places particular emphasis on improving the accessibility of mainstream schools and ensuring continuity of care and equality of opportunity as young people approach the transition to adulthood.

Wales has a similar programme to *Quality Protects*, called *Children First*. There is no Scottish equivalent as yet, although the Scottish Executive is 'committed to developing' a childcare strategy for Scotland, aimed at children aged 0–14, which 'delivers in each neighbourhood quality childcare services which are affordable and accessible' (Scottish Executive 2001). However, there is little specific mention of disabled children. The review of services to people with learning disabilities in Scotland (Scottish Executive 2000) made a number of recommendations which apply to children, for example, the appointment of local area co-ordinators, each working with a small number of families to co-ordinate services, information and funding.

Very little policy attention has been paid to the needs of siblings. Although the English, Scottish and Northern Irish legislation is broadly similar, a key difference is that the Children (Scotland) Act includes children 'adversely affected by the disability of any other family member' as 'children in need'. This may be aimed primarily at children with disabled parents (especially 'young carers') but includes brothers and sisters of disabled children (although it should not be assumed that all are 'adversely affected'). At practice level, there is some small-scale direct work with siblings across the UK, usually in groups, giving them a chance to share their views and experiences and offer mutual support where needed (Tozer 1996).

The research background

A great deal of research has been carried out about the effects on the family of caring for a disabled child. Many of the early studies adopted a patho-logical approach, taking the view that 'a handicapped child makes a handicapped family' (McCormack 1978). Indeed, where parents have reported beneficial effects of having a disabled child, these have sometimes been dismissed as evidence of denial or an attempt to alleviate guilt (Stainton and Besser 1998). Stainton and Besser are unusual in having looked at the positive impact disabled children can have on family life. Overall, however, the findings of many studies appear to conflict, making it hard to draw clear conclusions.

More recently, attention has been paid to the ways in which parents actively respond to and manage the various demands they face. Beresford (1994) examined parents' coping strategies, concluding that service delivery should be tailored to fit into and enhance these. A high level of unmet need for support among parents, children and siblings has frequently been identified, as has dissatisfaction among parents with service delivery and co-ordination (Russell 1996a). Baldwin and Carlisle (1994), reviewing the literature on social support for families with disabled children, point out that while numerous support needs have been identified for all the family, these have invariably been inferred from parents and professionals, and not from children.

Research on siblings' views

Relatively little research has been conducted about the siblings of disabled children. Baldwin and Carlisle (1994) suggested that much previous research on siblings was based on the assumption that they experienced psychologically damaging effects as a result of having a disabled brother or sister. These authors argued that actual evidence about emotional and behavioural problems in siblings was sparse and often based on methodologically dubious studies. Stainton and Besser (1998) found a more 'balanced' view in recent studies, but with a focus on siblings' 'functioning'. Some parents perceive their non-disabled children as more mature and independent than they might otherwise be (Glendinning 1983) or more altruistic and responsible (Tozer 1996). Parents have reported that siblings require information and explanations about the disabled child's condition and in some cases genetic counselling (Baldwin and Carlisle 1994).

Few researchers have talked directly to siblings of disabled children. Those that have done so report either mixed effects (NCH Action for Children 1995; Tozer 1996; Waters 1996) or mostly positive ones (Mackaskill 1985). For example, in a survey of 24 siblings of children with Prader-Willi syndrome (a rare genetic condition present from birth), positive comments were made about the individuals' 'loving, funny, caring and kind' personality, willingness to help others, sense of humour and a view that their presence had brought the family closer. Difficult aspects included having to deal with poor prognoses, being unable to do things spontaneously as a family and coping with stubborn behaviour and temper tantrums.

Mackaskill (1985) interviewed young people, aged 9 to 25, whose parents had adopted children with learning difficulties. Despite their initial apprehensions, these siblings were said to view the disabled children as 'unique personalities whose presence radiated family life'. Only 2 of the 22 siblings in this sample reported negative reactions. The others focused on the child's 'quirks and charms'. Most had no trouble saying what the child was good at; some had difficulty thinking what s/he could not do. Similarly, Lobato (1990) reports that young children, asked to describe their disabled sibling, did not mention impairment.

Thus, research suggests that growing up with a disabled brother or sister brings rewards and difficulties. The balance between these may have as much to do with the circumstances of individual families and parental coping styles as with the nature of impairment (Tozer 1996). Beresford *et al.* (1996), reviewing the literature on 'what works' in services for families with disabled children, report that findings about the effects of demographic characteristics, gender, birth order, family composition and characteristics of the disabled child are inconclusive. They suggest that more dynamic variables, such as family relationships and maternal depression, are more significant in determining the impact of a disabled child on her/his siblings. The authors conclude that while siblings are at increased risk of developing behavioural or emotional problems, there is considerable variation in individual response.

It is important to place the findings about siblings of disabled children within the wider literature on siblings. Lobato (1990) suggests that fighting and hostility occur between the most affectionate of siblings and that the ability to love and defend, despite some feelings of hostility and anger, is unique to sibling relationships. A study of the views of 69 primary school children about their siblings found that the latter were seen as a significant source of support and help, and that this was especially true where a child had few other supportive relationships (Kosonen 1996). Some problematic aspects of the relationships were also reported: siblings could be annoying, dominating and even abusive, particularly when left in charge of a younger child. Morrow (1998), interviewing non-disabled children aged 8–14, found that sibling relationships, while important, were rarely conflict-free, but underpinned by mutual affection and support.

Research seeking the views of disabled children

Like the research on families with disabled children, studies focusing on the disabled child have often taken a pathological approach. The main point of interest has tended to be how far the children were able to adapt, psychologically and emotionally, to what was assumed to be a personal tragedy with far-reaching negative consequences – the presence of impairment. However, Baldwin and Carlisle (1994), in their literature review, found evidence that some children do 'adapt and cope well'. They concluded that while many children are very unhappy and have not found ways of coping, significant numbers do attain 'normal' goals, have a good self-image and a sense of control over their lives.

However, most of this research was, again, based on parents' or professionals' accounts. Very few talked to the young people themselves. Baldwin and Carlisle did not find any study which had focused in detail on disabled children's daily lives and their views of the impact of disability. There had been virtually no research into these children's feelings about how they are treated by others, be it professionals or their non-disabled peers. Little was known about the experience of being disabled from the child's point of view and what makes it better or worse.

In recent years, considerable attention has been directed at seeking the views of children generally. A number of books and papers have appeared discussing methodological and ethical dimensions (e.g. Alderson 1995; Hazel 1996; Williamson and Butler 1995). Most of these do not refer to disabled children. However, a few texts have been published recently outlining ways to include disabled children in research. Minkes *et al.* (1994), Ash *et al.* (1996) and Morris (1998b) outline methods they have used in particular studies; Cavet (1995) interviewed a number of researchers about methods they had employed to include disabled children while Beresford (1997) and Ward (1997) have produced more general texts based on literature reviews. Other examples include Children and Society (1997), Children in Scotland (2000) and Potter and Whittaker (2001).

Ward (1999) brings together some conclusions from a programme of research about services to disabled children funded by the Joseph Rowntree Foundation. She concludes that disabled children's 'fundamental human rights' (such as the right to be consulted) are often ignored, especially where they have high support needs and/or communication difficulties. Nevertheless, it is evident that disabled children have opinions and feelings which they are well able to communicate, if asked in an appropriate way (Morris 1999). (See for example Abbot, Morris and Ward 2001; Anderson 1997; Kelly, McColgan and Scally 2000; Morris 1998a, 1998b, 1999, 2001; Noyes 1999; Stone 2001.)

Most of these studies have focused on children's views of services and support. It is still rare for research to take a broader approach, asking children about their wider life experiences and aspirations, although a few have. Flynn and Hirst (1992), who spoke to 79 teenagers and young

people with learning difficulties, present a sombre picture. Although there were exceptions, the majority of these young people led segregated and isolated lives, with young women facing particular disadvantage. There was little evidence to suggest that social participation or personal independence increased with age. Yet at the same time, these young people had very similar interests and aspirations to non-disabled people of the same age. These findings contrast with those of Laybourn and Cutting (1996) who interviewed 21 young people with epilepsy. They reported that the majority coped well and were 'positive and active'. Most received significant help from their parents and had good relationships with their peers.

Robinson and Stalker (1998), who edited a book about 'growing up with disability', initially sought to bring together the findings of research with a focus on the child's perspective. However, it soon became clear that many aspects of this topic remained unexplored. To begin to address these issues, some new work was commissioned for this collection. Certain recurring themes emerged:

- the taunting and bullying faced by many disabled children both in mainstream and special schools
- the centrality of the child's relationships with parents, especially mothers
- the experience of being treated as 'normal' within the family may or may not be empowering
- the need for services to take a holistic family and social model approach
- the importance to children of being asked for their opinions and being listened to
- the fact that children's views can be very different from those of their parents.

One study which has explored the everyday lives of disabled children from their own point of view is that by Watson *et al.* (2000). This research, part of an ESRC research programme entitled *Children 5–16: Growing into the twenty-first century*, was an ethnographic study of children aged between 11

and 16, aiming to explore their perspective on life as a disabled child. The authors found a diverse range of experiences, and responses to experience, among these children. Far from being passive victims, many were said to feel 'happy and successful'. Nevertheless, bullying again emerged as a central theme in their lives. The authors conclude that where children did experience difficulty, this was often as a consequence of social barriers to participation such as poor physical access, the attitudes of others or the isolation imposed by attending a special school outside their neighbourhood.

Models of disability and childhood

This study draws on insights and ideas from two fields: disability studies and the sociology of childhood. Disability has been defined in many different ways over the years; not surprisingly, these definitions have been influenced by varying historical, social and ideological practices. For many years, professional policy and practice has been dominated by the 'medical model', which equates disability with chronic illness, ascribes a 'sick role' to the individual and focuses on physical dysfunction (Oliver 1990). People are classified and defined in terms of their particular diagnosis or condition. It is often assumed that the person will have an adverse psychological response to having an impairment and that the professionals' job is either to 'cure' the problem (e.g. by cochlear implants or prosthetic limbs) and/or help the individual 'adjust' to their circumstances. The medical model underlies some of the literature cited above.

Closely allied to this perspective is the 'personal tragedy' model (Hevey 1993). Here, the experience of being or becoming disabled is assumed to be a continuing personal tragedy, and it is up to the individual to adjust to the tragedy and to society (Oliver 1993). Some people may be seen as having outstanding success in overcoming the odds against them, thus attaining the status of 'hero'.

In contrast, the social model of disability draws a distinction between *impairment*, meaning a physical, sensory or intellectual limitation and *disability*, which refers to the social, material and cultural barriers which exclude disabled people from mainstream life (Abberley 1987; Finkelstein 1980; Oliver 1990). Oliver argues that, during the rise of Western indus-

trialism, disabled people came to be seen as an economic burden because they were unable to undertake the heavy physical labour required in factories and mines at that time. They were subjected to harsh regimes in workhouses, thus creating an enforced dependency which, Oliver argues, still exists today. The social model has had a far-reaching impact on the way disabled adults are seen and see themselves. However, disability studies have shown little interest in the perspectives of children with impairments or the potential relevance of the social model to children's lives.

Until recently, much research on childhood was concerned with children's psychological, physical and social development. Children were generally ascribed a relatively passive role in this process (Waksler 1991) and viewed through adult eyes. This perspective underlies much of the literature on disabled children discussed above. In contrast, the 'new sociology' of childhood views the institution of childhood, unlike biological immaturity, as a social construction influenced by factors such as class, gender and ethnicity. Children are recognised as having a unique perspective and being active in shaping their own lives (James 1993; James and Prout 1997). With the increased interest in children's own accounts of their experience has come an acknowledgement that their lives are not homogeneous and need to be studied in all their diversity (Brannen and O'Brien 1995). Thus, micro-level accounts of children's lives – their life stories, their personal experiences – are essential for any macro-level analysis of childhood in general.

However, reliance on personal experience, so prevalent in the field of childhood research, is a contested area within disability studies. Indeed, some commentators (Finkelstein 1996; Oliver 1996) question whether it has any relevance at all:

> over a period of time, the political and cultural vision inspired by the new focus on dismantling the real disabling barriers 'out there' has been pro-gressively eroded and turned inward into contemplative and abstract concerns about subjective experiences of the disabling world. (Finkelstein 1996, p.34)

The concern here is that any attempt on the part of disabled people to describe the detail of their lives is simply a route back to viewing disability as a tragic event which 'happens' to some individuals.

A contrasting view is provided by a number of disabled feminists (Crow 1996; Morris 1993, 1996; Thomas 1999). They suggest that for personal experience to be relegated to the 'private' sphere and have no relevance in the public (and therefore political) domain is to ignore lessons from the feminist movement:

> In opposition to Finkelstein's view that a focus on individual lives and experiences fails to enable us to understand (and thus to challenge) the socio-structural, I would agree with those who see life history accounts … as evidence that 'the micro' is constitutive of the 'macro'. Experiential narratives offer a route in to understanding the 'socio-structural'. (Thomas 1999, p.78)

Thomas is one commentator who has been developing definitions of disability which relate directly to the experience of people's lives. She views disability as being rooted in a social relationship – an unequal social relationship. It follows a similar course to racism and sexism and results in the 'social imposition of restrictions of activity on impaired people' by non-impaired people. Her definition of disability has a further strand: 'disability is a form of social oppression involving the social imposition of restrictions of activity on people with impairments and the socially engendered undermining of their psycho-emotional well-being' (Thomas 1999, p.60).

For Thomas, any definition of disability has to include a psycho-emotional dimension, that is, the effects of being stared at, pointed at, hurt by the reactions of others, being made to feel worthless, of lesser value or unattractive. This aspect of disablism also arises from oppressive relationships – in other words, those social barriers which restrict 'being' as opposed to 'doing'. 'Psycho-emotional' is not to be confused with the 'psychological problems' attributed to disabled people by some sections of the medical profession but strongly challenged by disabled academics (Finkelstein and French 1993; Shakespeare and Watson 1997). Rather, it is an attempt to highlight an area of disablism[1] 'which is little explored within disability studies but evident when disabled people describe their lives.

The significance of impairment is also being re-evaluated in disability studies. A number of authors, including Crow (1996), Morris (1996) and Thomas (1999) note the presence of 'impairment effects', that is, restrictions of activity which result from living with an impairment. Thomas uses herself as an example: she does not have a left hand and the fact that she is unable to hold an implement in that hand is an effect of her impairment. This *impairment effect* may, however, become a conduit for *disability*. If someone decided that, since Thomas is unable to hold things in her left hand, she is unfit to do a particular job and should be denied employment, then 'the disability resides in the denial of rights' (Thomas 1999). In her opinion, one of the great political strengths of viewing disability in terms of an unequal social relationship is that it becomes possible to separate disability from impairment effects and thereby challenge the notion that all restrictions of activity are the result of the 'tragedy' of impairment.

The notion of difference underlies another debate relevant to this study. Generally, difference is viewed in two distinct ways by disabled academics. The first view is that it does not exist and is socially constructed: that is, individuals' bodies are constructed and then maintained as disabled by the opinions and barriers which exist within society (Price and Shildrick 1998). The alternative view is that disabled people can be seen as 'essentially' different from non-disabled people (Thomas 1999), so that difference is part of the 'essence' of a disabled person. Morris (1991) is a particular proponent of this approach. For her, having an impairment makes one fundamentally different from those who do not have impairments. This difference exists over and above the socially constructed effects of disablism, making the presence of an impairment the key difference between disabled and non-disabled people. Thus, for Morris, the difference which results from impairment is more significant and far-reaching than difference produced by other variables such as gender or age.

Possible links between the two quite separate fields of childhood sociology and disability studies are explored by Shakespeare and Watson

(1998). They argue that bringing together ideas and understandings from these two areas offers a fruitful way forward for exploring disabled childhood. At the same time, they caution that an awareness of the isolation experienced by many disabled children should not lead into seeing them as tragic victims; that a perception of disabled children as a social group should be balanced with the knowledge that they are also diverse individuals; that, while understanding similarities, we must remain alert to the differences, including those relating to class, race and the implications of specific impairments. Dowling and Dolan (2001) argue that a social model perspective highlights the way in which not only the child with impairment, but also the whole family, can be disabled by unequal opportunities and social barriers.

The fusion of ideas from disability studies and the sociology of childhood may, as yet, be an uneasy marriage – or an early courtship – but with the growing endorsement of 'the personal' in disability studies, there are at least some common strands which can provide a framework for this research. For example, Thomas's work (1999) sits well with the idea of using micro-level accounts to support macro-level analysis: the idea that disability exists within the context of an unequal relationship will be used as a backdrop to analyse the accounts of disabled children and their families in the following pages. Her contention that the disablism which arises out of this unequal relationship can affect not only what people do, but also who they are – their sense of self – will inform discussion about the children's understanding of disability. Finally, care will be taken throughout the chapters to ensure that impairment effects are noted so that the extent to which disabled children have to contend with social barriers is clarified, without losing sight of the role that impairment may also play. To ignore such effects would be to deny the diversity and richness of children's experiences and important details about their everyday lives.

Notes

1. Thomas defines 'disablism' as 'exclusionary and oppressive practices at the interpersonal, organisational, cultural and socio-structural levels in particular societal contexts' (1999, p.40).

Chapter Two

Conducting the Research

Introduction

This chapter describes how the study was carried out, including how we gained informed consent, designed the interview materials, communicated with the children and involved two young people as advisors to the project. It ends with a brief description of the disabled children's characteristics and circumstances. More detail is given about methods than is sometimes the case because of the growing interest in how to conduct research with disabled children, and seeking their views more generally.

Methodological approach

In order to explore the children's perceptions in depth and with sensitivity, a qualitative approach was adopted. This methodology involves exploring the world of the participants, in order to describe and understand the social environment from their point of view. Qualitative studies are recognised as making a distinctive contribution to the sociology of childhood because they enable children's voices to be heard more directly. As already discussed, there has been an upsurge of interest in children's own accounts of their lives, along with an understanding that these lives are very complex (Brannen and O' Brien 1995). Qualitative approaches have been used increasingly in disability studies (Morris 1996; Thomas 1999), as the details of disabled people's lives are explored.

It was also decided that the study should have a participatory element – two young disabled people were involved in the initial design. There is a

growing literature on the participatory paradigm in relation to disabled people (Cocks and Cockran 1995; Oliver 1992, 1993; Ward and Flynn 1994; Zarb 1992). This approach is based on a number of ideas. First, conventional research relationships, with the researcher as 'expert' and the researched merely the object of investigation, are inequitable and fail to recognise the extent to which expertise resides in the research participant. Second, people have a right to be involved in research which is concerned with issues affecting their lives. Third, the quality and relevance of research is improved when disabled people are involved in the process.

Previous research exploring disabled children's perspectives on their lives has focused on 11 to 16 year olds (Watson *et al.* 2000) or older teenagers (Hirst and Baldwin 1994), leaving a significant gap in relation to younger disabled children. It was important to include boys and girls (Flynn and Hirst 1992), having found that young women with learning impairments were more socially isolated than their male counterparts. We wanted to include children living in rural areas, towns and a city, services to disabled people being considerably less developed in rural areas (Stalker and Reddish 1995) and to involve some children in residential schools, since this group is particularly disadvantaged on a number of levels (Abbot, Morris and Ward 2001; Morris 1995).

Recruiting children and families

The original intention was to contact parents through local education authorities, to avoid any bias which might arise through recruiting children from social work, health authorities or parents' organisations. Although some families were recruited through schools, this approach had limited success, with several head teachers declining to pass on information about the research to parents. Some believed families were under particular stress and did not wish to 'bother' them. Others thought our study, with its focus on disabled children, was contrary to their policy of inclusion. Where schools did pass on information to parents, the response rate was low. Subsequent approaches to a number of voluntary organisations working with disabled children and their families proved more effective.

In both cases, parents were initially sent a letter about the research, written by the researchers but signed by a professional known to the family, inviting them to take part and enclosing a reply slip. Following a positive response, the researchers sent agreement forms to the children, as described below. Eventually 25 families were recruited, with 26 disabled children, 24 siblings and 38 parents taking part. Although the sample was not selected to be representative of the wider population of families with disabled children, the children did have the range of characteristics, in terms of age, gender, location and type of school, that we aimed to achieve.

Informed consent

In recent years, increasing attention has been paid to the concept of informed consent and how best to obtain it. Beresford (1997), Ward (1997) and Alderson (1995) discuss this in relation to disabled children. Informed consent is closely tied to the notion of 'competence' and is said to comprise three elements: understanding, wisdom and freedom/autonomy (Bersoff and Hofer 1990). Competence can be assessed in three ways: by status, function and outcome (Brazier and Lobjoit 1991). However, consent is an ambiguous concept, the more so when children are involved. Macklin (1992) suggests it might be more appropriate to seek consent from parents and 'assent' from children; this was the approach used in this study.

With parental consent, agreement forms were sent to the children. These were colourful, illustrated leaflets addressed personally to each child, containing a photograph of the researcher who would be visiting the family and setting out, in simple and concrete terms, the purpose of the study and what participation would involve. There were two versions for disabled children: one for those aged 8–10 (see Appendix A), another for 11–14-year-olds (see Appendix B). Two agreement forms were designed for siblings, aimed at the same age groups (see Appendices C and D). All the forms stressed confidentiality and the willingness of the researcher to use the child's preferred communication method. At the end of the project, children would receive a booklet telling them what we had found. The forms included a section to be signed either by or on behalf of the child to signify her/his willingness to be involved in the research.

Gaining initial consent from the children was, however, only part of a continuing process. Each time the researcher and child met, it was emphasised that s/he could end the interview at any time or even pull out of the project – it was entirely their choice. For the most part, the children were more than willing to be involved. However, one young disabled child who had been happy to attend the first interview was clearly disgruntled when he arrived for the second. When reminded that he was free to say he did not want to be interviewed, this boy opted to go out to play instead. He later decided to leave the project. Another young disabled child signed his agreement form but withdrew his consent before the first interview and did not take part in the project. However, his parents and older sibling were interviewed. Several siblings declined to sign the agreement form and so were not included in the interviews. These incidents were both frustrating and gratifying for the researchers – frustrating, because they denied the project valuable data, gratifying in that they suggested children felt able to give and withhold consent freely.

Two children, one from the older group and one from the younger, had complex support needs. It was not possible to gain informed consent nor interview either child directly but the researcher requested time to observe the children, having established with the parents that at any sign of discomfort or distress on the part of the child, the observation would stop immediately.

Visiting the families

A series of visits was then made to each family in their own home. The whole family was invited to attend. The aim was to discuss various issues in more detail than had been possible through the agreement forms, notably:

- purpose of the research
- topics to be covered
- length of visits
- willingness of everyone to participate
- permission to tape record

- confidentiality
- dissemination of the outcomes of the research.

This visit was also an opportunity for family members to 'check out' the researcher and allow her, in turn, to gauge the children's level of ability and methods of communication so that suitable materials were used in subsequent visits. We told families we hoped to talk with children and parents separately, to enable both parties to speak freely and allow differing opinions to emerge. One of the older children requested that his mother be present throughout the interviews. Siblings could choose whether to be interviewed alone or together.

Following the initial visit, most disabled children were interviewed twice, although two had an additional visit. Parents and siblings were each interviewed once. The visits to each family were usually completed within a fortnight. With one exception, all the interviews took place in the family home. Interviews with the disabled children and siblings ranged from 40 minutes to an hour or more. Parental interviews could take up to two hours.

The interview schedules and activities

The schedules were piloted with five families (these interviews were included in the main sample as very few changes were made). Older disabled children were interviewed using a topic guide, while younger ones and those with learning impairments had a more structured schedule covering the same topics (see Appendices E and F). Prior to each interview, the younger children were offered the opportunity to produce drawings, make a tape, or write about people or things that were important to them: any materials which they produced were used as a 'warm up' for the interview. If no materials were forthcoming, the researcher took a little time with the child to reflect on what had been happening in her/his life since the last visit.

The schedules for younger disabled children and those with learning difficulties included various questions in conventional format. For example, children were asked what they did on a typical school day and at the weekend. Visual aids, activities and games were also used, partly to

engage the children's interest and make the interviews 'fun', partly to facilitate communication with children who had cognitive, hearing or communication impairments. For example, 'spidergrams' were used to ask the child about important people in her/his life (see Appendix G), and things s/he worried about, and 'lifelines' to help her/him identify 'good' and 'bad' things which had happened (see Appendix H). Questions about favourite activities were accompanied by picture cards, as were those about professionals and services. In a 'word choice' exercise, children were presented with a brightly coloured A4 sheet showing four rows of three words each. They were asked to circle all the words which described what they were like at school, for example, 'happy', 'fed-up', 'friendly', 'lazy' and 'sad' (see Appendix I).

To explore themes of independence and inclusion, the children were asked to construct a 'neighbourhood map'. They were given a metal board with magnetic pictorial counters depicting various landmarks such as 'my house', 'school', 'shops', 'park', 'church', 'swimming pool' and 'library'. Children were asked to draw a map of their neighbourhood by placing these counters on the board, and to talk about when and why they would, or would not, visit these places.

Children were seldom asked directly about their impairment. We did not wish to make it a bigger issue in their lives than it perhaps was. Rather, we wanted them to describe and delineate its impact. However, if a child consistently did not refer to their impairment, we used supplementary questions to raise the topic.

The topic guide for older children covered the same areas as the schedule for younger ones but most questions were worded differently. Older children were not usually asked to do exercises, unless they seemed to be 'stuck' on a topic. Similarly, interview schedules were designed for 'younger' (see Appendix J) and 'older' siblings, the former including some pictorial materials and activities (see Appendix K). All the children gave permission for their interviews to be taped.

Communicating with the children

Great care was taken when working with disabled children and their siblings to ensure that appropriate language and communication methods were used. Four of the children communicated in sign, using either British Sign Language (BSL) or Makaton, which is a signing system derived from BSL but adapted for use by people with learning difficulties. Makaton employs facial expression and sometimes symbols and is always accompanied by speech. The children using these communication methods were interviewed by one of the authors who has fluent sign language skills. The interviews conducted in BSL were video taped. A number of other children had significant speech and language impairments so parents were consulted about ways to adapt materials and the appropriateness of the language the researcher intended to use. In these instances, the researcher took detailed notes of the interviews to supplement the recordings. Two of the children preferred to engage with written materials; in one case, all the interview materials were re-written in book form with the child himself as the main character.

Another child, with autistic spectrum disorder, used facilitated communication. His mother worked through some of the interview schedules with him using a home-made board containing all the letters of the alphabet and a few basic words such as 'yes' and 'no' (their usual method of communication). She would take her son's hand and he guided her to different letters, gradually making up words and sentences. This enabled the inclusion of a child who would otherwise have been excluded from the study. Facilitated communication remains controversial, however (see Mostert 2001 for a review). Where, later in the book, we quote data from this boy, we alert the reader that these were obtained through facilitated communication.

To help children with reduced vision, picture cards were produced with matt rather than gloss surfaces. Where children could not read or write, due to visual or cognitive impairment, the researcher did so for them. Further detailed discussion about the interview process and communicating with the children can be found in Stalker and Connors (2002).

After the interviews

When the interviews were completed, each child was sent a thank-you card and a small gift. Those who had requested copies of their taped interviews received them shortly afterwards. Families were kept informed about the progress of the study via a series of newsletters.

To analyse the material, audio and video taped interviews were transcribed in full; the transcripts were carefully read several times and analysed manually. Emerging patterns, common themes and key points were identified and these, together with additional material taken from field notes and pen profiles of the families, were used to distil the findings. In writing this book, we have used as much information as possible from the children themselves, drawing on parental interviews mainly to clarify issues when appropriate or to highlight contradictory views where they exist.

Project advisors

Two disabled children (aged 11 and 12) acted as study advisors. They were contacted through Enlighten, a voluntary organisation in Edinburgh, which provides support for people with epilepsy. The girls were involved in three meetings about the project and gave valuable advice, particularly about the research proposal, the children's agreement forms and the interview materials.

Description of the sample

Fifteen boys and 11 girls took part in the project, reflecting the higher incidence of impairment among males in the general population (OPCS 1989). They were aged between 7 and 15, the largest group being 9- and 10-year-olds, of whom there were 13. One child of mixed race took part in the study. The rest of the children were white, reflecting the relatively low incidence of ethnic minority families in most parts of Scotland. We deliberately avoided using a medical definition of 'disability' as a criterion for inclusion in the study. Thus, the children had a variety of impairments – learning, sensory and physical. Thirteen had learning impairments, five had sensory impairments and six physical. As already indicated, two

children had complex support needs (see glossary for definition) and a number had dual impairments.

The disabled children were being educated in a variety of settings. The highest proportion, 12, were in segregated settings (special schools) with nine educated inclusively (mainstream schools) and five in integrated settings (units attached to mainstream schools). One boy attended residential school. By the end of our fieldwork period, all the children in the older age group, bar one, were being educated in segregated schools. Of the 25 families who took part in the project, six were single parent and four, step parent. There were four only children in the study. Information about siblings can be found in Chapter 6. The families were located across central and southern Scotland: six lived in cities, 16 in towns and three in rural communities.

Summary

The study used a qualitative approach and included a small participatory element. Despite some difficulties recruiting families, 26 disabled children with a range of characteristics, 24 siblings and 38 parents took part in the research. Wherever possible, consent was sought from children: throughout the interview process they were reminded that they were free to withdraw if and when they chose. Different materials were used for older and younger children, and data collection was adapted as appropriate for children with sensory, cognitive and communication impairments.

Chapter Three

Children Negotiating Day to Day Life at Home

Introduction

This chapter presents the disabled children's accounts of their everyday lives at home and in the wider community. It begins by looking at their overall attitude to life and sense of achievement therein. It then discusses their relationships with family and friends and inclusion in the wider community. The main focus of the chapter is on the 'ordinariness' of the children's lives and how social barriers, including psycho-emotional ones, intrude upon this. The following chapter looks in more detail at their experiences in school.

Attitude to life

Achievements and difficulties

All except two of the children interviewed were able to name at least one thing they were 'good at'. Some did so in consultation with their parents. These can be divided into successes inside and outside school. Outside school, the children's achievements straddled a wide variety of activities including:

- athletics
- swimming
- football

- gymnastics
- wrestling
- horse riding
- using a computer
- dancing
- drawing
- singing
- cooking
- doing jigsaws
- riding a bike.

The prevalence of achievement through sport should be noted. Several children talked about winning medals for various sporting activities, working towards awards in particular sports and the pleasure of being included in a team. One older girl had just won a place in the Olympic squad for swimming and athletics. A younger boy said he was good at everything – 'I'm the best'. Other children, however, described less lofty achievements. An older boy reported he was good at 'pretending' while another believed himself to be 'very good at playing'! A younger boy was unable to think of anything he was good at – everything at school was 'hard' and although he had won a medal for football at a summer playscheme, he did not link this with being skilful.

The children were also asked to name something which they found difficult. Six children could not think of anything. Two mentioned physical things such as not being able to drink juice when it was too 'tangy', while the largest number of children immediately related the question to school and began to describe difficulties in particular subjects. The other children were either unable or unwilling to answer the question, so information was sought from parents.

Here, a very different picture emerges. Parents of children with autistic spectrum disorder talked about the difficulty for their children of any change in routine. One mother of a ten-year-old boy explained: 'The minute the sameness goes, then Kenny's anxiety levels go up.' This anxiety

would manifest itself as either aggressive behaviour or extreme distress which could only be ameliorated by making Kenny's world predictable again. Another child had great difficulty coping with other local children calling him names. His mother believed people did not understand this could upset him: '…that he's just, he is just a mongol and that he is a spassi and that you don't have to worry about upsetting him because that's all he is.'

There seemed to be a very different 'feel' to the perception of difficulty in children's and parental accounts. For most children, things which presented them with difficulties were concrete and, it would seem, experienced on a daily basis. The struggle to learn times tables, doing spelling homework, writing a story, all have an immediacy which is not reflected in parental interviews. Parents give more evidence of occasions when either their child was excluded or when people behaved in hurtful, inappropriate ways towards her/him or, indeed, towards the parents themselves. The children seem to be less concerned with focusing on such incidents. Closs (1998) suggests it would be wrong to assume that children share parental perspectives and warns that the child's view may be lost as parents struggle to manage their own feelings of frustration and loss, particularly as they compare their own and their child's experiences with that of others. However, later in the interviews, some older children recounted experiencing hurtful reactions from other people and some described being bullied, corresponding to Thomas's (1999) psycho-emotional facets of disability. Some children also expressed frustration with restrictions to their social lives: for Thomas, these restrictions would be examples of barriers to 'doing'. Both are discussed in more detail later, but it is interesting that the children did not, apparently, think of these experiences when asked about things they found difficult.

Making choices

The children were asked if they had enough say about what happened in their day to day lives. The younger children and those with learning impairments were invited to complete a 'Choices Chart' which looked at the pattern of everyday choices they made, while the older group was invited to comment on the level of choice they had in their lives. All the

children made some choices for themselves. For those with complex support needs, making a choice was actively encouraged as part of their daily routines. Similarly, one of the girls with autistic spectrum disorder was being encouraged to use choice more, especially in relation to food. For the majority, the main choices they made were to do with after-school activities and whom they played with. Some children made choices about what they wore, though for the most part these were shared decisions with parents, as were decisions about what time they got up, what happened at weekends and on birthdays and what food they ate.

There was evidence of some older children either taking increasing responsibility for their lives or working hard to be allowed to do so. One 14-year-old boy felt he made all his choices for himself: 'No, people don't make decisions for me. I do it myself.' A parent of a 12-year-old boy with a learning impairment made a link between her son's choices and his happiness: 'He chooses what he wants to do, he does it and it makes him happy.' Some older children were involved in choices about their schooling. One 14-year-old boy described his reasons for choosing to go to a particular school: 'Well, all my friends and everything were all going up there so I decided I wanted to go too.'

Most young people felt they had enough say in what happened in their lives. Two wanted more choice: one girl wanted her mother to let her wear track-suit trousers to school and one of the boys wanted more choice about whom he played with. His mother did not like some of his friends so he was unable to play with them at home.

Feelings of happiness and sadness

Twenty-three of the 26 children involved in the study were asked how often they felt happy: most, some or none of the time? They were also asked what made them feel happy and what made them feel sad. Most children declared themselves to be happy most of the time, with some feeling happy 'all of the time'. Happiness was linked to general experiences such as being with friends or family, achieving things, going on holiday and playing games or sports. For the children who deemed themselves to be happy most (as opposed to all) of the time, feelings of sadness were usually related to specific events. These included the illness or death

of a relative, being bullied in school or bored at home, and arguments with family or friends. Those children who described themselves as being bored at home contrasted this with having plenty to do at school. One older child described being 'stuck in the house on a Sunday' and the feelings of boredom and frustration that brought.

Of the remaining children interviewed, one talked about being happy some of the time: asked what would make her feel happy for more of the time, she replied 'If I could walk'. She was in the process of recovering from a major operation related to her impairment. One older boy declined to answer the question. Three children were not interviewed; one of the younger group had decided against it. The two children with complex support needs were able to communicate happiness and sadness to their families and those who knew them well. Their parents felt these children were happy most of the time.

Relationships

With parents

When asked to identify important people in their lives, the majority of children interviewed named either their mother, or their mother and father, as very important. There were many examples of close, loving relationships between disabled children and their parents. When asked why mother/parents were so important, some of the children replied thus:

> Because they help me.
>
> 'Cos they're there for me.
>
> Because I love them very much and they help me…they look after me.
>
> 'Cos she's the best.
>
> Because I'm grateful, because they give me everything.
>
> They give me telly, computer, CDs, videos…

Receiving help and support from parents is a strong theme through many of the children's interviews: they described spending time with their parents, playing with them, going out to places and doing things together. Two of the children, however, did not mention parents at all among the

important people in their lives. They chose to concentrate on friends instead. The ambivalence some children feel towards their parents is also reflected in the work of Thomas (1998) and Closs (1998).

Closeness between disabled children and their parents may not always have positive outcomes. Bignall and Butt (2000), researching the views of young black disabled people about living independently, noted that family support could often restrict young people's ability to be independent because the family wanted to 'protect' them. Several of the children in this study, two of them with physical impairments, described not being able to visit local friends because their parents would not allow them to cross a busy road. This had the direct result of restricting their friendships and for one girl in particular, it meant she was not able to spend time with her only local friend. A mother of a child with a learning impairment recognised that the desire within herself to protect her ten-year-old son might not always be in his best interests:

> It's more me that I can't take that step. I don't feel he's fit to do that at the moment, you know. I couldn't let him out with other children of ten year old. I don't feel they're responsible enough because they just treat him like one of themselves. They could turn away and be doing something else and Danny could wander off, you know.

This mother acknowledged a positive aspect to the fact that other boys treated Danny exactly like themselves. However, fears for his safety led her to intrude upon their relationship and insist that friends came to play with him at his house. This reduced both his number of friends and the activities they could do. Danny also spent long periods playing alone at home. Not all parents were over-protective. A few of the disabled children were encouraged to go to the local shops on errands for their parents, as were some of the young people in Bignall and Butt's study (2000). This was viewed as a sign of 'growing up'. For example, one boy, having reached his ninth birthday, was now deemed mature enough to go to the local shop on his own.

A number of the older children with physical impairments had issues around gaining independence whilst still having to rely on their parents, notably their mothers, for a high level of physical care. For example, 13-year-old Lorna described how her days began with a decision about

breakfast. This decision, though small, was a sign of her determination to be more grown up:

> So then my mum shouts me and I come down for my breakfast whenever I want because she's treating me like an adult now. 'Cos she didn't realise that I'm growing up and treats me like a five-year-old.

This was a theme throughout Lorna's interviews. Her talk of growing up contrasted with the language her mother used to describe her, referring to her daughter, in the interview, as a 'little girl'. Lorna was working hard to challenge this assumption:

> She's got to understand that she can't rule my life any more. Because when I get older she's just going to tell me what to do but I just want to make up my own mind because she's always deciding for me, like what's best for me and sometimes I get angry. She just doesn't realise that I'm grown up now but soon I'm going to be 14, in September, and I won't be a wee girl anymore.

Having a carer who was independent of the family went some way to alleviating the situation. This carer, who came to help in the evenings, usually took Lorna and her cousin bowling twice a week. The carer also enabled Lorna to make her own decisions about when she bathed and went to bed. However, Lorna still had to rely on her mother for help in the mornings. One of the older boys was asked about receiving care from his parents:

Interviewer:	Do you think the relationship with your mum and dad differs from if you'd been able bodied?
Child:	It would be different because they have to lift me.
Interviewer:	So does that make a difference your mum and dad doing physical things for you? For someone your age?
Child:	Yes.
Interviewer:	What way does it make it different?
Child:	Don't know what to say.

His mother also identified this as a difficulty, particularly since her son's condition was degenerative and increasing levels of care were likely to be needed:

> ...it's hard for both of us because you've got a relationship where at this age Peter should be sort of looking for his autonomy and his identity and moving away and he, he needs me, you know. He needs me to brush his teeth, to put his deodorant on, he can't say to me 'Oh piss off' and slam the door. I've got to slam the door for him...

With siblings

Using questions on a colourful illustrated sheet (see Appendix L), younger children and those with learning impairments were asked to describe the best and worst things about their siblings, when they had fun, when they got on together and when they annoyed each other; older children were asked more general questions. Most of the young people said their sisters and/or brothers were very important to them. Three did not mention their siblings when talking about 'important people', including the two who did not identify their parents as important. Children and their siblings seemed to get on best and have most fun when they were playing together, involved in a wide variety of activities including football, playing with dolls, playing cards, going on holidays and wrestling.

As with all sibling relationships, there was evidence of conflict too. Most of this conflict revolved around arguments caused by incidents such as toys being taken, siblings not listening or being 'nasty'. Four of the younger children believed they never annoyed their siblings and thus did nothing to cause any of the conflicts in which they became embroiled. Others recognised their own role in the proceedings. One girl said of her relationship with her sister: 'I'm annoying her, she's annoying me.'

Three children felt their siblings bullied them. One younger child reported being bullied by his two brothers who were a number of years younger than him. This 'bullying' took the form of pinching and scratching him and taking toys from his room. The two other children talked about more violent incidents with their siblings. A boy from the younger group described his relationship with his older brother in terms of being punched, kicked and 'whacked'. This brother was described by his parents as having challenging behaviour himself. When the younger boy was asked why his brother might behave in this way, he replied: 'Because he's a bully and he likes it.' A younger girl also described being physically attacked by her older brother. As with the boy above, she never played with her brother. However, both of these children had more positive relationships with younger siblings in the family. A number of other children described being closer to one sibling, or preferring the company of one sibling to another. The boy with autistic spectrum disorder, who used facilitated communication, described his confusion about relating to his sisters at all.

There was evidence of disabled children helping their siblings and being helped by them. Two of the disabled children, the oldest in their family, talked about helping their younger siblings in the mornings. One of these boys talked about having chats with his little sister about 'what it's like to get bigger'. In turn, some siblings were helpful to their disabled sister or brother. In some cases this was a general helpfulness, while other children gave particular examples. One girl described being taken on walks by her elder brother; a teenage boy said his older sister was a useful source of information about 'girl/boy' relationships and he had no hesitation in discussing such things with her. There were, however, suggestions that indiscriminate helping was not welcomed by some disabled children. One boy became annoyed when his sister tried to help without his permission: 'I know she's trying to help but if I'm doing something and I don't need her I shout.' Another boy was unhappy with his older sister always being around him: '...she bugs me at home. I'm always telling her to stop it but she keeps on...'

The picture which emerged when disabled children talked about their relationships with siblings was one of complexity and diversity. There was little evidence of a group of passive children, around whom the family revolved, being ministered to by their siblings. Rather, there were suggestions of some robust relationships with fun and conflict in equal measure, reflecting the pattern of sibling relationships in the wider literature. In a few cases it would appear there was a great deal of conflict, some of it violent, with siblings, notably with older siblings. This is discussed from the siblings' point of view in Chapter 6.

With the extended family

Only four disabled children identified extended family members (two aunts, an uncle and maternal grandparents) as important to them. It is clear from the interviews, however, that children had frequent contact with their extended families, many of whom lived nearby. Four children detailed much of their social life as involving cousins, aunts and uncles. An older girl described a number of family parties she had attended, while a boy from the younger group talked of regular outings with his cousins. Nine children made regular visits to grandparents. One child mentioned visits from an uncle and four had an aunt to whom they were close: one of these acted as a carer for the child on a regular basis.

Despite regular contact with extended families, a number of parents felt unsupported by them. There were various reasons for this, notably, that extended families viewed the disabled child as 'different' and were unsure how to treat her/him. This lack of confidence resulted in either withdrawal or inappropriate behaviour and was a frequent source of upset for a number of the parents. One parent talked about her extended family wanting to exclude her disabled daughter: 'It was actually my brother who said, "Could she not be put in respite for the wedding?" And they asked Joanne (her sister) to be bridesmaid but not Marie and that's just because she's disabled.' However, none of the children indicated an awareness of hostile attitudes from extended family members.

In a number of cases, relatives provided short breaks for the children from their parents. This will be explored in more detail in Chapter 5.

With friends

Most of the children interviewed identified at least one friend who was very important to them, with 'playing together' the most frequent reason for friendship. Two predictors of friendship pattern emerged: the type of school a child attended and her/his parents' attitudes. Watson *et al.* (2000) note that children who travelled to schools located a distance away from their homes, either because they were attending segregated (special) schools or because their local mainstream school was not accessible, had few friends in their local community. They tended to socialise with family members instead. A similar pattern is present here. Seven of the children

who attended either segregated schools or were in integrated (unit) settings to which they had to travel daily, seemed to have no local friends. They reported feelings of boredom when not at school and four of them relied on family members for a social life. The other three children seemed not to have a social life at all. As one nine-year-old boy said when asked about his life outside school: 'I just sit and watch cartoons on the couch.'

A 13-year-old girl sometimes went out on Saturday with a family member but after that:

Child:	...I just watch telly and then I go upstairs and play with the playstation.
Interviewer:	And on Sundays?
Child:	On Sundays I just watch Hollyoaks and the Waltons and I play on my computer...I'm just bored.

There were, of course, exceptions to the dominant pattern. One boy, who attended a unit for part of his day and was in mainstream for the rest, talked about a variety of local friends. A teenager who had moved from a local mainstream to a special school further away still felt closer to his friends at home:

It's like weird because people at my school, they are not as much my friends as people here 'cos I don't know them that much. My friends past the years, they come to my house but not them. They've never even seen my house.

One of the younger boys, who had no school friends in the area, told of a close friendship with a boy living at the end of his road: he had taught his friend sign language and they were able to communicate with each other. However, as his mother pointed out: 'He doesn't have as many friends as he would have had if he was in a primary school class with 30 children.' Another older boy, who attended a segregated school, named a number of local friends whom his mother said were younger than him. She was concerned, too, that some of them may have been bullying him.

Disabled children in inclusive (mainstream) settings seemed to fare better. All but one had several local friends with whom they would meet up either after school or at weekends. Most of these friends attended the same

school as the child and were usually, but not always, in the same class. Shared activities included attending clubs, bike riding, playing football and forming a band. It should be noted, however, that all except one of these children were of primary school age while those in segregated settings were mostly of secondary school age. Indeed, some of the latter initially attended local primary schools where, according to their parents, they did have local friends. Most of these friendships seem not to have withstood the transition to a different school, suggesting that friendships currently enjoyed by the younger children may be at risk in the future.

The other factor affecting disabled children's friendships seems to be the ability of their parents to allow them the freedom to be with friends. This point has already been illustrated in relation to parental roles in promoting children's independence, but there are a number of other examples. One of the children aged nine, who attended an inclusive school, was said by his parents to have no local friends. Although this boy would invite a number of friends round to his house (sometimes without the agreement of his parents), his mother described them as 'too active for Robbie'; they would want to go and play football and he, who was less active, would be left behind. During the course of the interview, however, other possible reasons came to light:

> Like we say to him 'You will need to stay here' or 'You can only go as far as'...that's for his own safety. He finds things like that quite hard really, because he sees other kids and, of course, other kids are running about so eventually they do go away and he is left on his own and quite often you look out and he's standing there on his own...we try to let him go out without us being there, we watch him all the time but he used to, for a while, just go and we would look out and he'd be gone and we're panicking.

Adult surveillance seems not to be compatible with the development of child friendships. Some parents seemed to recognise this and accepted that their disabled child had to form relationships outside the family, even if this entailed some risk – children playing outside, going off on bike rides, going beyond adult view. Other parents, however, appeared to want to give their child's friendships careful boundaries. In these cases, friends were invited to the house (thereby limiting the activities they could do),

children were expected to play in certain areas or were encouraged to play within the family, notably with much younger siblings or members of the extended family. Watson *et al.* (2000) note the high levels of adult surveillance in the lives of disabled children as a whole.

Negotiating the wider community

As discussed above, many of the children's outings to places like shops and parks took place in the company of adults. However, some children did frequent their local parks, go to nearby shops and explore their neighbourhood without their parents. One mother described how her 13-year-old son, a wheelchair user, and his friends would go to the local shops:

> He's always been treated age appropriately...when they all had skateboards, when they were younger they would go on the skateboard, they would hold on and the ones that had roller blades too and he would pull them along and Kevin (his friend) stands on the back of his chair, to go along to the shops.

Interests

There was great similarity between the things children felt that they were good at and their interests. Interest and a sense of achievement seemed to go hand in hand. There was, however, a clear gender divide in the children's choices. Interests for the boys were mostly sporting and/or outdoors activities such as football, wrestling, riding bikes, climbing trees, snooker, darts, bowling and watching videos. The girls pursued a more diverse mixture of sports and home-based activities, including swimming, bowling, athletics, dancing, drawing, using computers, watching videos and listening to music. Music was very important to the two girls with complex support needs. The mother of one of them described the perseverance necessary to encourage her daughter to listen to music:

> I started off (with the phonic ear) and Karen really, really didn't like it. It was such a new experience and you know, you just touched her ears with the mould and she...oh. So it started off with just seconds, then minutes over a very long period of time...and built it up and built it up over a very long period of time with lots and lots of touch or using music and sounds and now it's a really key part of her life.

Boys who wanted to pursue their interest in football also had to be persevering. Most managed to play football in school and some, with friends at home. The children did not minimise the challenges of playing football with non-disabled peers. Apart from practical difficulties such as wheelchairs getting stuck in wet grass, there was also the issue of being included in the game at all:

Child: But I hardly get a touch of the ball.

Interviewer: Oh, why is that?

Child: It's probably just because I'm in a wheelchair.

The same nine-year-old still had moments of triumph: 'I played for my school team and I scored a goal.' Another boy's talents were almost missed because he attended a unit attached to the school and did not get to play football with boys in the main school during the day. When his skills were eventually recognised, he was given a place in the school team.

If the boys wanted to take their football any further, however, and a number of them expressed a desire to be a professional footballer when they grew up, the only option open to them, even if they used wheelchairs, was a mainstream football team. The children did not seem to view their impairments as barriers to full participation: one nine-year-old boy had written to his local adult team requesting that he join and explaining he would have to play using his walking frame. However, there was no evidence of any football teams for children with physical impairments nor, indeed, of any attempts to introduce sporting role models for the children.

The overwhelming interest in football by the boys did not seem to be matched by a similar interest in any one thing among the girls.

Clubs and playschemes

Children were involved in a variety of clubs and organised activities outside school, including Brownies, Cubs, sports and youth clubs. Anna was ten years old and lived in a city. On Mondays she went to a line dancing class at the local deaf club, on Tuesdays she attended Girls' Brigade and on Wednesdays, went swimming. On Saturday mornings, she had a gymnastics lesson at her local sports centre. Like many young

children, then, Anna had a busy week attending a variety of activities. Unlike most children, however, at least one of these activities was segregated. Some children expressed a preference for being with their non-disabled peers. A 14-year-old boy, who complained about the inaccessibility of his local youth club, wanted all clubs to be inclusive and all disabled people able to join in: 'I think it would be better if they could join in with everyone else because they should be treated the same as everyone else and do the same things.'

There was particular difficulty for children who lived in rural areas. One boy had been declined a place at his local youth club, on the grounds that it could not 'cope' with his impairment but, because he lived in a small village and his family did not own a car, this really meant he was excluded from most of the social life for children in his community. He spent a lot of time watching television. Another boy living in a rural area relied on his mother or grandmother to take him to and from any activities in which he was involved.

Playschemes were often something of a mixed blessing. They were usually temporary and run at specific times during the year. Those which were run by voluntary agencies, specifically for disabled children, were trying to cater for a wide range of needs and in some cases met very few of them. One boy attended a scheme run by a voluntary organisation only to find he was having to mix with children who had very different needs from his own; another boy was taken to places which were not accessible. When children joined local authority playschemes, there did not seem to be any attempt to ensure their requirements were met. No sign language interpretation was available for a boy with a hearing impairment when he attended a football scheme. Written notes and drawings were used to communicate with him and while he was happy to take part and obviously enjoyed the experience, no real thought had been given as to how to include him.

It is striking that, as children grew older, there was less for them to do. This may be a reflection of the fact that, in adolescence, other interests come to the fore or it could be an indication of the paucity of activities on offer to older children. There is evidence in the literature (Cheston 1994; Thomson et al. 1995) that, as children grow older, physical barriers become more apparent. Young people tend to move from an organised form of leisure to a more casual one (Cavet 1998): they gather in settings like fast food outlets which are difficult for young disabled people to access (Watson *et al.* 2000). Simon, aged 13, liked to go shopping with his friends at the weekend. The shopping centre had Shopmobility (wheelchairs provided for use by disabled people for the duration of their shopping), however, the wheelchairs available were for adults, not for children, so moving around the shops was difficult for him. Simon and his family sometimes went out for a meal. He found it embarrassing having to be carried up steps into a restaurant and wondered why people had to stare: 'I don't mind if it's wee boys or wee girls that look at me but if it's adults…they should know. It's as if they've never seen a wheelchair before and they have, eh.'

Summary

Overall, the disabled children reported that they were happy, good at a variety of things, had friends and, for the most part, felt they had enough say about what happened in their lives. Most were close to their parents and siblings. There was a degree of conflict between some disabled children and their brothers and sisters, as would be expected between most siblings. Many children had regular contact with their extended family. Some parents encouraged independence in their disabled children while others adopted a more cautious and protective approach, which could have the effect of limiting the young people's activities and restricting their friendships. The type of school that children attended also affected the friendships they developed, with those at special schools or units outside their neighbourhood usually having few friends locally.

The children had a variety of interests. Many of the boys were very keen on watching and playing football but opportunities for the latter were limited, especially for those with a physical impairment. Girls tended to enjoy sports and home-based activities. Younger disabled children were more likely to attend clubs and playschemes than older children, with some evidence that teenagers were excluded from a number of age appropriate gathering places and activities.

These findings can be related to Thomas's definitions of impairment and disability discussed in the previous chapter. The children identified (not in so many words, of course) certain impairment effects, such as a lack of, or restricted, mobility. They also referred to a number of barriers they faced in everyday life. Thomas argues that impairment effects can become a conduit for disability, leading to socially imposed restrictions on activity. Examples evident from the young people's accounts include inaccessible buildings, inaccessible transport and a lack of appropriate support for communication, all of which affected their ability to pursue age appropriate pastimes. However, the children seemed perhaps more concerned by attacks on what Thomas would call their psycho-emotional well-being, such as name calling and bullying. It is noticeable that some parents reported similar experiences, for example, through the hurtful remarks or behaviour of relatives. These themes will be explored in more detail in later chapters.

Chapter Four

Children Negotiating Day to Day Life at School

Introduction

This chapter presents the children's accounts of their experiences at school. They were asked to describe their school day in some detail, starting from the time they got up and finishing with when they went to bed. The first part of the chapter is an overview of the children's feelings about school. This is followed by a closer look at their experiences in segregated, integrated and inclusive schools. The final section is about bullying.

Attitudes to school

Most children interviewed were positive about school: 'It's brilliant, being at school is better than being at home, I enjoy most things in school.' Two children, whilst having positive things to say about being in school, also had ambivalent feelings. These were mostly to do with finding the work either boring or a struggle to do: one child found the act of writing a problem, the other talked about his difficulties with literacy. Three children were quite clear about their dislike of school. One nine-year-old boy summed up his feelings: 'I wish I could do that, stay off school and just watch the telly.' Again, this boy expressed a dislike of writing, which was physically difficult for him and meant he was frequently behind with his work. The remaining two children did not enjoy the particular school they were attending. The boy using facilitated communication described his desire to move to another school because he felt his needs were not being met in the unit where he was placed. The following extract is from a letter he wrote, through his mother, to the head teacher. The boy gave permission for the letter to be passed on to us:

> I am feeling very frustrated and annoyed as a result of attitudes to Facilitated Communication. I feel able to avail myself on a level of education far beyond what your school is providing me at the moment. I believe that I need an education more suited to my needs.

The other boy who expressed unhappiness with his school placement was attending a residential special school. He was clear about his dislike of this school but very positive about his experience in an inclusive school which he had attended for a number of years before moving first to a special school (which he also disliked), and then to residential school. His mother, who was present at the interview, requested a copy of the interview tape to give to his children's rights officer.

As described in Chapter 2, the children were invited to complete an exercise choosing positive and/or negative words to describe themselves at school (see Appendix I). They each selected at least three, usually more, positive words. The most frequently used word was 'helpful', followed by 'keen', 'happy', 'jokey', 'friendly' and 'sporty'. Children reported giving help to other pupils, their friends or their teachers. For example, one ten-year-old girl described how she was often sent to other classes with messages. She liked this responsibility and tried to be as helpful to other people in the school as they were to her: she especially liked to help the younger pupils. The children's choice of words in this exercise is particularly interesting in that it suggests a great deal of agency on their part. It seems they perceived themselves, in school, as being as much able to help other people as they are helped, as being good friends to others, good fun to be with and active. All this points to a very different picture from the pathologised/medicalised vision of disabled children's lives presented in some of the literature. It was also quite different from the views a number of parents had about their child's behaviour at school.

Among the less positive words on offer, the most frequently chosen were 'bored', 'fed-up' and 'sad'. As with the feelings of sadness described earlier, these seemed to be linked to specific, immediate events. For example, one of the older children talked about being fed-up in school, the day he was interviewed, because his two friends had had an argument and he felt caught in the middle. One of the younger boys was fed-up because another boy in his class had called him a name. His response was to tell his teacher and thereby ensure that the other child got a detention. The same pattern seemed to occur with the children who talked about being sad in school. Feelings of sadness were linked to specific events – one boy was sad that his friend had just been suspended, while a girl was sad that she could not take her favourite CD to school with her. On both these occasions 'sad' may have been used instead of a more graphic term! Boredom, however, was a more general feeling, with one of the children 'always' being bored in school and the others bored 'sometimes'.

Segregated settings

Twelve children attended segregated schools but only ten were interviewed, as this sub-sample included the two girls with complex support needs. It also included the boy at residential school. The fact that the other segregated schools were all impairment specific may explain a striking feature of these children's accounts. This group, more than children who attended inclusive schools or integrated units, talked about their impairments without direct questions or prompts from the interviewers. Indeed, two of the children were quite clear about wanting to attend their school because of their impairment: 'The only reason I like going to my school is because of my wheelchair.' Another young person had this exchange with the interviewer:

Interviewer:	You want to go to a school where there are lots of deaf children?
Child:	Yes…where there's signing, where everyone signs, all the teachers, all the children.
Interviewer:	Why is that better than going to a school with hearing children?
Child:	Hearing children – no-one signs. I don't understand them and they don't understand me.

One of the older boys described how children in his school were further segregated according to their impairment:

Child: Well, there's all the walking people round because hardly any of the wheelchair people can get in there.

Interviewer: And are they referred to as walking people?

Child: The walkers, that's what they call them.

Interviewer: Who calls them that?

Child: Every single teacher.

Interviewer: What do they call you then?

Child: The wheelchairs, but it's the person inside the wheelchair
                that counts, not the chair that counts.

Similarly, one of the older girls said: 'I'm happy being a cerebral palsy.' There has to be speculation about how such a self definition could come about. Was it a consequence of being referred to over a period of time as 'a cerebral palsy', in the same way that some children were apparently referred to as 'a walker' or 'a wheelchair'? These two children attended the same school: was this way of describing them peculiar to that establishment? Watson et al. (2000) also found that some teachers categorised and labelled children, even going so far as to introduce them to visitors, in terms of their impairment. Davis and Watson (2001) add that the children were expected to comply with the definitions – and the accompanying status – imposed on them by teachers. The effect on children's self worth – or their psycho-emotional well-being (Thomas 1999) – of such definitions is not clear from this example. It does suggest, however, that the medical model of disability, with its focus on type of impairment and limitations of function rather than seeing the child as a person, remains dominant in some schools.

In spite of this, the children in segregated schools reported positive feelings, for the most part, about their schools and their teachers. Initially, one boy said that he 'hated' all his teachers but later corrected this to some being 'alright' and disliking others. Tom was a 14-year-old boy who, having attended a mainstream primary, had the option of going to an inclusive high school but not the one his friends were going to, which was inaccessible for wheelchair users. He decided to opt for a segregated school instead. Tom was also concerned about being bullied in mainstream school. When asked to imagine himself still with an impairment but able to walk, attending the same school as his friends, he expressed worries about being 'shoved' down the stairs. In his view, the type of 'disability' a young person had should be a major factor in deciding whether to go to a segregated or inclusive school. Although Tom enjoyed some subjects, he said he was not worried that he would be taking fewer standard grades in his present school than he would have done in an inclusive school. There was little point in taking any exams or trying to get into college, he said, because 'no-one wants to employ disabled people anyway'. Similar comments about the non-academic orientation of special schools have been made by disabled people elsewhere (People First Scotland 1996).

All the children interviewed named friends in school, though several commented on the difficulty of seeing them in the evenings and at weekends. As one girl said: 'I get a good education and people are looking out for me and that. My friends, that's the difficult part...I don't see them a lot...' One evening a week there was a youth club at Tom's school. His local authority would not provide transport and suggested he waited in school from the end of lessons until the start of the youth club. However, Tom was unwilling to hang around from 3.00pm until 7.00pm, nor was he happy about not being able to change out of his school uniform to go to the club. Another special school had plans to create after-school clubs and a third had instituted an after-school award scheme to provide the children with some kind of social activity in the evenings.

Integrated settings

Five boys, but no girls, were attending integrated units. All took part in some interviews, although this group included three unusual interviews: the child who used facilitated communication, the boy for whom materials were rewritten in book form and the child who withdrew after the first interview. Two were in secondary placements – in fact one of these boys had moved from a special school to a unit. He was the only child in the study to move out of a segregated school. The other boys were in primary units. None of these units were in the children's local communities so they had to travel to and from school in taxis or buses. As mentioned earlier, two of them reported having no local friends. None described taking part in any after-school activities which may, again, have had something to do with a lack of transport to and from events.

Only one of the boys talked about spending part of his day in the main school and part in the unit. The mother of another boy reported that her son did spend some time within the main school but how much time was not clear. According to this parent, the quality of the integration had to be questioned anyway because:

> ...the head teacher seems to have no idea about, you know, the fact what integration is all about. He has not sort of taught any of the mainstream classroom teachers anything about autism. I think they had half a day at the beginning when the unit was opening...and they've had nothing since...it's up to the teacher if they want to allow a child with autism into their mainstream classroom, it's up to them.

The remaining children spent their days in the unit and so were, in effect, in a segregated setting. Two of these children reported close friendships with other children in their unit. Finally, one of the older boys was spending his school day on his own, with two members of staff. His mother explained how this happened:

> ...it is a very sociable event being with other children. But he's segregated from other children. Now he's not even, he never sees his class. He doesn't spend any time in his classroom, never...that wasn't what I wanted for him...it's all down to resources...he needs one to one on his Record of Needs.

This boy was due to move to a segregated school at the end of the current term, a move which had been suggested to his parents shortly after he began in the school, aged six. He was 12 at the time of the interviews. According to his parents, the head teacher was not happy having him spend more time with his class. It was felt that the 'gap' between him and his peers was 'widening' to an unacceptable level. The role of professionals in the success or failure of disabled children's placement in inclusive and integrated settings will be discussed further in Chapter 5.

All the children in integrated settings who were interviewed spoke positively about their teachers and believed them to be very helpful. One boy expressed annoyance that his 'special needs' teacher was often away on training courses and they were left with a supply teacher whom he considered to be less good.

Inclusive settings

Nine children were attending inclusive schools. Seven of these were at their local primary school and one at high school, though this child was in the process of arranging to be moved to a segregated school. Eight of the nine were interviewed. Their accounts illustrate the diversity of experience which a mainstream school offers disabled children. For example, all had some kind of learning support with much variety in how this was offered. In fact, it could be argued that the level and amount of support offered had much to do with the type of impairment a child had. All those with physical impairments had a full time helper at school – a post which seems to have a number of titles, including 'special needs assistant' and 'learning support worker'. Children with sensory impairments were visited by a specialist teacher. These visits could range from an hour a week to an hour a day, but in other cases only took place when specialist equipment was required.

For children with learning impairments, the picture was even more complex. Some worked in a particular group where support, in the form of either a teacher or an assistant, was shared with a number of other children; others were withdrawn from their class for a time each day or once a week. Whatever the model of support offered to children with learning impairments, a number of parents felt it was inadequate. One mother of a ten-year-old boy described it thus:

> …they tell you if you ask for anything special that, oh well, that's a lot on the budget and for one child. They refuse to, they refuse to recognise your child as being one of a (number of) special needs within the school. They single them out as being 'the special needs child' who's going to require all these resources and all this extra input. But, I mean, we have a

full time learning support at the school and she does not have enough time for all the children...she's only two periods a week with George. So where does all the rest of her time come?

The children often had mixed feelings about the support they received. A few described assistants as very helpful but some children with a full time helper were more ambivalent. For example, one of the younger girls was very annoyed with her helper for taking her to a different playground, where younger children played, away from her friends. Despite parental complaints to the head teacher, this had not been addressed. Davis and Watson (2001) comment of disabled children in 'inclusive' settings: 'Their opportunities to be fully included in the same social spaces as other children were restricted because many learning support staff and educational psychologists did not take account of sub-cultural relationships between children' (p.675).

A number of parents also had questions about the appropriateness of the behaviour of their child's assistant. The mother of a 14-year-old boy reported her son's regular complaints about his assistant:

> Like she'll go up and she'll like kiss him and she sings to him... she does all sorts of childish things...he's already asked, you know, for her to go and for another person to come and it was really hard for him to do that. But they said, no, we can't really sack her for caring too much about Roy.

This mother also felt that the presence of an assistant had an inhibiting effect on her son's relationships in school. Shaw (1998) found similar concerns among disabled children with special needs assistants. This issue is discussed in more detail in Chapter 5.

The children in primary schools were all positive about their teachers, including one boy who did not like school. For the young man in high school, some of the teachers were 'fine' and others clearly not. He particularly liked his Home Economics teacher: 'She just treats me like everyone else.' However, another of his teachers had a very different approach: 'Well, one of my teachers, he talks to my helper but he doesn't talk to me and that's quite annoying...if he talked to me instead of my helper that would be better.' He was still deciding how best to deal with this teacher.

Bullying

Watson *et al.* (2000) reported that disabled children endured widespread bullying: many felt that bullying was the one thing all disabled children had in common. Almost half the disabled children interviewed in this study said they had been bullied. Seven had been bullied in school: as already discussed, two were bullied at home by siblings and a further two children were bullied by others in their locality. One boy experienced bullying both in school and by children who lived around him. Bullying in school took a number of forms, including name calling, excluding the child or not talking to her/him, extracting money and, occasionally, physical violence. It took place in all three types of setting although, within this small sample, only girls were bullied in segregated schools. In many cases bullying seemed to be an isolated event which, once dealt with, did not reoccur but for a few children it was a regular experience. One boy described how frequently he was bullied:

Child: When people bully me and make fun of me.

Interviewer: And how often is that?

Child: About nearly every day.

Interviewer: What do you do?

Child: Go and tell the teachers.

Interviewer: Uhuh, and what do they do?

Child: They give them detention for it.

Interviewer: And does that help?

Child: A little bit.

This bullying seemed to be linked to the child's impairment: his mother reported that he once said he had had a good day in school because no-one had called him 'blindie'. Despite some very creative work by his teacher to help the other children understand his impairment, the bullying continued.

Other children were more successful in their attempts to deal with bullying. Their strategies had been to tell their parents or a teacher, or to take direct action themselves. When children chose the first option,

schools soon got to know about it. Some were slow to act and it took persistence on the part of parents to have action taken. For example, Paul, aged nine, had 'lots of friends in school' but some time ago, had become 'fed-up' because some of his friends stopped talking to him. He was not sure why this happened but his parents believed it was because Paul had been kept back a year while his friends moved on to the next class. At first, Paul's school did not accept there was any problem and told his parents not to worry. However, they insisted that Paul was being teased and was unhappy and, eventually, the school took action to stop the teasing. Consequently the situation was resolved, with Paul now having friends in his new class as well as keeping some from his old class. One of the older girls who was being bullied decided not to approach teachers for help. With the support of her mother, she faced the bullies in her special school and was not bothered by them again.

There is evidence from elsewhere of children in special schools bullying as well as being bullied (Watson *et al.* 2000). In this sample, the mother of a 13-year-old boy identified his bullying behaviour and the possible reasons for it:

> ...he'd always been the lowest in the pecking order in mainstream. And when he went there was him and another boy – the two most intelligent in the class, way, streets ahead of everybody else because they'd been in mainstream. Em and Liam decided that he felt the kingpin and he was a bully and I was horrified...I think that for once in his life Liam felt powerful.

There was no evidence from children or their parents that those who were in inclusive schools or units were acting as bullies.

For the child who was bullied both at school and by children in his local community, the bullying took different forms. In school, bullies were extracting money from him but, once the problem was recognised by his mother and reported to staff, it was managed and did not recur. As he played outside at home, however, he was repeatedly subjected to name calling. His mother reported his distress at such treatment but seemed to have no strategies for dealing with it.

Summary

Most children enjoyed school and were positive about their teacher. Indeed, some enjoyed being at school better than being at home because they had more to do. Some parents whose children were placed in integrated settings questioned the amount, and quality, of time their sons spent in 'the mainstream', although the children themselves did not mention this. Children attending special schools talked more openly than others about their impairment. Some felt that their school suited their particular needs well. However, there was evidence of at least one such school focusing on impairment in a less than positive way, encouraging the children to define themselves in this way. Children attending inclusive schools received a variety of levels and forms of support, although some had mixed, or negative, feelings about the role of special needs assistants. Those attending schools outside their neighbourhood had less contact with school friends outside school hours and/or fewer friends locally, than did those at local schools. Some children had been bullied in school; most had strategies for dealing with this and once dealt with, bullying did not recur. However, for others, bullying was part of their daily life.

Again, these findings can be related to Thomas's notions of impairment and disability. It is striking that the children identified few impairment effects in relation to their schooling, although a lack of dexterity and difficulties with literacy were mentioned. More evident in this chapter are the disabling barriers they faced, in terms of inaccessible transport and buildings, school policies on segregation, integration and inclusion and, in one instance, lack of support for communication. Despite some feelings of frustration, to a large extent the children seemed to accept these obstacles. Again, it was the bullying and teasing experienced by some children which had a more immediate and distressing impact – hardly surprising, given the 'in your face' nature of name calling or exclusion. The discrimination caused by a lack of accessible transport or being called a 'wheelchair' may be less obvious to some children, particularly younger ones, if that is what they have always known, if such practices appear to be sanctioned or carried out by adults, or if they feel there is little they can do to change structural barriers. However, it must be emphasised that unhappy experiences were reported by a minority of children. There was considerably

more evidence of the young people having positive self-images, of being active agents and dealing with any difficulties with resilience and initiative.

Chapter Five

Services and Professionals

Introduction

This chapter examines disabled children's experiences with services and professionals. It looks at what families had to say about health, education and social work services, finishing with a discussion about short-term breaks for children. The disabled children were asked about the helpfulness or otherwise of doctors, nurses, teachers, and social workers (should they have one). They were also asked to describe any experiences they may have had in hospital, in a short breaks facility and attending clubs or playschemes. They were asked about any other people who helped them. All the children interviewed were able to comment on their teachers and, in some cases, helpers, and most were able to comment on either a GP or a consultant. Only one child spoke about her contact with a social work professional. Other professionals identified by children were physiotherapists, occupational therapists, a community care worker and a children's rights officer.

Nevertheless, in this chapter more than in any other, we draw on parents' accounts of their sons' and daughters' experiences, for the interesting reason that the young people themselves had relatively little to say on this topic. At the same time, we have excluded quite a number of the comments made by parents, on the grounds that these were often more about their own views and experiences, rather than the children's. This is not to say that parents' experiences, and their responses to those experiences, are not valid in themselves; however, the focus of this book is on the

children. Many other studies have explored, and largely confined themselves to, parents' views about services.

Parents' accounts differed from the children's in the range and tone of the experiences they described. While the children were, for the most part, positive about the professionals they encountered, parents were more qualified in their approval and very clear about what constituted good and bad practice. There was some evidence, however, that older children showed increasing discernment about the quality of services offered to them.

Health services and professionals

Hospitals

One of the most striking features of this sample is the frequency of contact most children had with health services. The medicalisation of impairment, well documented in disability studies (Priestly 1998), is evident here. Most contact was with hospitals, attended by 22 children, for reasons ranging from assessment and monitoring to post-operative (much of it elective) care.

STAYING IN HOSPITAL

Fifteen children had experience of one or more stays in hospital, usually, but not always, involving surgery. Parents used a range of approaches to prepare children for going into hospital. Some explained the process in detail, others felt that such explanation would only lead to increased worry for the child. The mother of an eight-year-old boy felt it would distress him to know too much about his impending surgery:

> Because a little information worried him. You know he's better going in and having whatever was done at the time because if I did tell him, 'Oh tomorrow they'll come and give you a jag in the morning and make you go to sleep', he would worry from the night before.

One hospital provided a booklet to help parents explain to children what a spell in hospital might entail. Others seemed to rely on doctors visiting the child and her/his parents for a pre-operative talk. One nine-year-old boy felt it was better to know all the information about his operation in advance: 'The doctor who was doing my operation came and told me everything that was going to happen.'

None of the children interviewed found being in hospital a particularly pleasant experience. Although parents were able to stay with them, it was often a difficult and painful time which, for one young man with a physical impairment, was made worse by a lack of appropriate facilities. He had to make regular trips to an adult ward on another floor to use an accessible toilet. This aside, the children were mostly positive about the doctors and nursing staff they encountered in hospitals. One of the older boys, however, reported that some professionals did not listen to his 'requirements'. He was regularly admitted to hospital on an emergency basis and found the staff tried to treat him in ways contrary to his wishes. However, he was happy to point this out to them: 'I usually have to give them a right earful before they listen to me, but I usually get my own way if I do that... it should be up to me because I'm old enough.'

Most parents felt that doctors in hospitals explained things to children clearly, using age appropriate language. On the whole, they talked directly to the children rather than the parents. However, difficulties could arise when children were admitted to teaching hospitals and subjected to a steady stream of doctors in training. One parent commented:

> So you get a lot of young doctors coming and asking you a hundred and one questions... That's happened where they've come and they've asked questions that Dougie is perfectly able to answer himself...like does he like juice...you know. Well ask him. And then you'll get the other ones that will come in...and they're speaking in real kind of medical jargon that I dinnae even understand.

OUT-PATIENT APPOINTMENTS

The majority of children interviewed had regular appointments in hospital clinics. This was not a difficult experience for most. Indeed, some of the doctors seemed to go out of their way to accommodate children's needs, particularly those with more severe impairments. One boy who found changes to his routine distressing was always seen by the same doctor, with the same nurse accompanying him in the same environment. When something more problematic had to be done, such as taking a blood sample, this

took place in another location so the boy would not associate his visit to the consultant with an unpleasant experience. This was one of several examples of potentially difficult situations being managed with creativity and sensitivity by medical personnel.

However, other doctors appeared to focus solely on the negative aspects of impairment and seemed not to be concerned about causing the child distress or making difficult situations worse. For example, one family had a difficult time at an Accident and Emergency (A&E) department following a problem which developed after their daughter had surgery:

> We took her to A & E and the member of staff who helped me, the health member of staff, refused to treat her, even though she was in agony, screaming in agony…he said he wasn't going to get involved because she already had a consultant and he wasn't that consultant and his quote was 'too many chiefs'.

These parents eventually received an apology from the hospital. They felt that had their daughter not had an impairment, she would not have been treated in this way.

Primary health care

For most children, visits to GPs were rare. The parents of the two girls with complex support needs chose to circumvent GPs altogether and dealt directly with a consultant or, in times of emergency, with a hospital. The boy at residential school had a GP some miles from home: he also saw a consultant in time of need.

While most of the children interviewed spoke well of their GP and perceived him or her as helpful, it was unclear if they were always sure who their GP actually was. In fact, it may be that some children were referring to the doctor they saw in hospital, since making the distinction was quite difficult. From parental accounts, however, it is clear that the children attended doctors' surgeries for minor ailments, on rare occasions. When it was necessary to take their child to a GP, some parents made a careful choice about which one to see:

> I only go to one GP if possible. We have to watch…not so much watch with the GPs… But there's about four of them down there who know

him over the years and who know his situation… They're very good, they really are.

The main reason for selecting a GP carefully was to avoid the need to rehearse the child's entire medical history. Also, parents felt that doctors who knew their child could manage recurring conditions more quickly.

Other health professionals

Six children were receiving physiotherapy, four had contact with an occupational therapist (OT) and three with a speech and language therapist. One child had input from all three. The children themselves commented mostly about their experiences of physiotherapists, while two boys talked about occupational therapists. The children's views about physiotherapy, and their relationships with physiotherapists, were mixed. One older girl recognised it was necessary if she wanted to keep herself mobile. An older boy felt he did not get enough physiotherapy and, if he had the funds, he would have more treatment to improve his mobility. However, he also expressed dissatisfaction with his present worker:

Child: For example, my physio. He sometimes goes a bit far, hurts me sometimes.

Interviewer: And what happens if you tell him?

Child: He says it's for my own good.

Interviewer: Right.

Child: But I think I should have a right to say how much he should do it.

The mother of this young man also had misgivings about the level and intensity of treatment her son was having to face. Her experience was that most physiotherapists knew little, if anything, about her son's condition and after treating him, would leave him in pain for a number of days. Most of all, physiotherapy was not fun: 'I would love to see somebody with the right attitude coming in and giving him a good going over and making it fun. It should have been fun from the word go.'

In contrast, one of the younger girls was enjoying her physiotherapy very much, mainly, her mother believed, because it was fun:

Oh yes, we like the physio, the hydrotherapy. Ken and Bob they are good fun. They throw her about in the water and splash and have fun so again she does enjoy it. If she doesn't think about what she's doing she is a bit better at doing things.

However, the mother of a ten-year-old boy described her son not being able to understand the language of professional assessments and thus, doing badly in assessment:

I found this with the physio…when he went in for assessment too. She used words that he wasn't used to so she wasn't getting the reaction that she was expecting, so she thought he didn't know. I says 'It's not that he doesn't know, he doesnie understand the word you're using because he uses a different word.'

The two children who mentioned OTs saw them as helpful. They could get hold of specialist equipment when it was needed and knew whom to talk to about adaptations to houses. A 14-year-old boy described the process:

She helped me a few years ago to get a toilet chair, a special one for me. And a bath chair that goes in my bath and straps me in. And she also got me a comfy chair to sit in if I'm watching the telly or something. So she was quite helpful… If you need anything…we just call her and she gets it for us.

However, there was little evidence of OTs taking a proactive role with children – staying in touch, monitoring what they might need, producing some kind of care plan – rather, although there were some exceptions, most appeared to work on an ad hoc basis, usually at the invitation of parents.

Both children and parents described the frustrations involved in getting certain types of equipment. There seemed to be particular difficulties with wheelchairs. One example was long delays between ordering a new chair and it arriving, which could mean that the child had outgrown the new wheelchair. Another was parents being told that, for cost reasons, they had to make a choice between having an electric chair or a manual one, even though their child needed both. Several parents commented on their incredulity that equipment which was central to their children's well-being was so difficult to acquire.

Although several parents talked about the frustrations involved in not having as much speech and language therapy for their children as they thought was needed, even when it formed part of the child's Record of Needs, none of the children commented on using this service.

Education services and professionals

Getting children into schools

As already discussed, the disabled children were mostly positive about school and school staff. Parents gave a very different view. Children who were, or had been, in inclusive schools made no mention of the problems some of their parents had encountered in securing and maintaining places in local schools: it was not clear if the children were aware of these difficulties. However, evidence of this 'struggle' (the word most frequently used by parents) is clear in many of the latter's accounts. In some cases, difficulties began as soon as parents decided they wanted a place for their child at a local school:

> It started right at the beginning when they refused to admit him, which was illegal and I pointed this out. And the head teacher had said, well, she had checked with her union and it was okay…to not register him unless he had the appropriate help. I says, well, I am fighting for the appropriate help and I'd like you to register him. But anyway, she didn't register him till the very last minute and by then I had called in my MP… I had to really, really fight.

This child had no learning support for his first year in school because resources had been given to another child, so sure was the school that he would not be accepted.

Other parents also found that head teachers played a crucial role in deciding whether or not to accept a pupil. Without a supportive head teacher, schooling for these parents became a series of battles round such issues as use of resources and the child's access to certain parts of the school. One mother described her struggle to get an appropriate special needs assistant for her daughter:

> Her special assistant left and at the time I was campaigning for SAs to have some kind of training to know how to handle kids with cerebral palsy. Any kid in a wheelchair needs to be handled correctly. So the head-

mistress employed an SA...just took her off the street...didn't know anything at all about Lucy...I had picked an SA for Lucy who was excellent...had all the training... The headmistress said no. So I just went above her head.

Not all parents had to fight to get their child into an inclusive setting. Two of the younger boys experienced no difficulties and were welcomed immediately by their local schools. Another younger child who began his education in his local primary school later moved to a segregated setting but not before the benefits of his presence in the school had been recognised. His mother believed that his being there encouraged the school staff to 'think in different ways' and to work as a team.

But, I mean, the head teacher's words to me at the end of it was, 'Mrs Smith, you think we've done so much for Neil, can I tell you that, no, what we've done for Neil is never going to measure what he's done for us.' And I think that said it all and it was said genuinely, you know.

Meeting children's needs

Those parents who did not meet opposition to their child's inclusion in a mainstream school still reported a certain apprehension on the part of schools and their staff about having a disabled child as a pupil. Parents had to tread carefully, over a number of years, to establish good working relationships with schools, sometimes weathering a variety of storms in their desire to have their child's needs met. Parents spoke of a number of problems around working with class teachers for whom a positive attitude about the child was essential:

...when I look back, em, the school had never had a deaf child and especially, a profoundly deaf child and I think they were very apprehensive about having Beth. And it was unfortunate that she had the same teacher in Primary 1 and 2 who wasn't my favourite teacher and I don't think she was particularly, em, she wasn't particularly welcoming about having Beth...we had a few difficult occasions with that teacher in that just, just her manner towards Beth perhaps was unfortunate at times.

This parent went on to report that having had a number of years with 'good' teachers, her daughter was making excellent progress and the school was more confident. The situation had also been helped by the presence of a specialist peripatetic teacher who encouraged the staff to work in partnership with parents.

As noted in the previous chapter, the involvement of a special needs assistant (SNA) was an on-going source of difficulty for some children. There is evidence from other research that disabled children spend a large proportion of their time in the company of adults (Watson *et al.* 2000) and certainly, the children with SNAs in this study seemed to reflect this. Both parents and children gave examples of these workers having an adverse effect on inclusion. In a number of cases, one of which was noted earlier, SNAs removed children from their peers at play and lunch times. One mother described the inhibiting effect an SNA had on her son:

> When he was at the age when they stick their tongue out at the teacher if she'd have her back to them, the SA was always with Jamie, so Jamie didn't get to do it. And other kids go here or there – Jamie was never allowed to go here or there and I found out that she was taking him into the nursery at lunch time to have his lunch, he'd be about eight, 'cos she was friendly with the nursery teachers.

In the previous chapter, children made it clear how much they enjoyed lunch and playtimes in school, yet the presence of an adult with a different agenda was reducing, or working against, these important opportunities for social interaction. It could be argued that in some cases the activities of SNAs created segregation in what should have been inclusive schooling.

Several parents also reported ways in which SNAs overstepped personal/professional boundaries and became over-involved in children's lives. One mother described how, when her son was ill, his SNA made repeated attempts to contact his family:

> But I mean when he was in hospital, it was cards every other day. She was phoning me at home, she found out my number and everything. She's really a bit over-anxious about him more than maybe he would like or maybe I would like...

Shaw (1998) stresses the importance of a high level of awareness and sensitivity in adults who support disabled children in inclusive schools. Skar and Taam (2001) conducted a study in Sweden exploring the views of 13 disabled children about their assistants. These assistants differ from those discussed above in that they may be employed by a statutory agency, a private company or by the user and they support children with personal care and social activities outside as well as within school. Nevertheless, the study findings are similar to those reported above. The children's relationships with their assistants are described as 'quite complex and ambivalent'. On the basis of children's reports, the authors identify five categories (p.923):

- the replaceable assistant
- the assistant as mother/father
- the professional assistant
- the assistant as a friend
- my ideal assistant.

Those who fell into the 'assistant as mother/father' category made decisions for the young people, seldom asked their opinion and treated them like 'children'. Such assistants were seen as 'an obstacle to their self-determination', for example, by taking over a play situation and deciding what or how the child was to play. The latter felt this discouraged other children from playing with them.

Despite the existence of inclusive educational policies for a number of years, parents' accounts suggest that many schools are not fully prepared to receive disabled children. There was a sense of each child having to break new ground, of parents having to insist that children had places in schools and that resources, allocated to meet their needs, were used appropriately. For the only boy in the sample attending mainstream secondary school, the desire to stay in the same school as his friends had to be balanced against the barriers he encountered on an almost daily basis in a school which, whilst happy to have him, seemed not to be in any hurry to provide the equipment he needed. He wanted to be the same as all the other pupils in the school but was repeatedly forced to be different, or reminded of his difference, by school practice. His mother commented on the disabling role of the school:

> I think it's always the same, it's access and equipment that Ron has the biggest fight with. They don't have the stuff for him... They don't realise what he's doing, you know, living with a wheelchair and it's not until you say 'Look, well what about this?' 'Oh yeah, this will take about two years

to get money for this...' I think every time he comes across it, it's the environment that makes him realise he's disabled.

Social work services and professionals

The 25 families who took part in the study had little formal or prolonged involvement with social work departments. Only four families had an allocated social worker and only one child chose to comment on this support, saying that she did not see much of her social worker. In two cases, parents expressed dissatisfaction with their current worker, one mother feeling there were no benefits to her daughter:

> She doesn't even have a relationship with the social worker. She doesn't have a relationship because she doesn't see her that often. I mean, if you were to say to her she was coming, she would say, 'Well, what does she want?'

The parents of a ten-year-old girl, who had recently been assigned a social worker, described their first meeting in not dissimilar terms:

> She came in and sat down and said 'What's going on? I have never done one of these before. I don't know what children's services are available in this area.' So she got handed a children's services document, a social work assessment one and she spoke to Fiona for a few minutes... You look to her for help and it's not forthcoming... I don't think Fiona would understand what a social worker is.

Another family described their social worker as making 'sympathetic noises' but not doing very much, although she had arranged short breaks for their son. The other family with an allocated social worker was subject to a different way of working. Here, contact was maintained through a children's rights officer who saw the disabled child regularly. The social worker involved had chosen to take a more managerial role and so had periodic meetings with the children's rights officer to keep abreast of the family situation. However, the child's mother wondered how the children's rights officer could be a truly independent advocate for her son when the social work department employed him.

Twenty-two families were without a social worker. In four cases this was a conscious decision, based either on a perceived stigma attached to

social work intervention, or on past experience of social workers express-
ing negative attitudes towards disabled children. One mother explained:

> One social worker said to us that we made the choice to have Julie at
> home so, and I said to her 'Well, how did I make that choice?', and she
> said 'You could have put her into residential care', and I said 'Well, I don't
> really think that is a choice.'

This mother felt that the family's 'choice' to keep their daughter at home
was seen by the social work department as absolving it from any responsibility. Two families wanted, but were having difficulty securing, an allocated social worker.

The majority of families had some contact with a social work department, either to arrange for their child to attend a local playscheme or, in a
few cases, to have a short break. One family had a very positive experience
with a nursery run by a social work department. Overall, however, there
was a clear feeling among parents that social work departments were slow
to act, not very helpful and usually not to be relied upon for any sustained
support.

Short breaks

Just under half the disabled children had some form of short break away
from their primary carer. While parents explained their use of short breaks
mainly in terms of creating more time for each other or for their other
children, a few also said that their disabled child needed and benefited
from time away from them. Several gave reasons for not using short-term
care; these did not include any objection on the child's part.

Short breaks seemed to follow a number of patterns for these children.
They took place in a variety of locations, as set out below. Some were
regular, planned breaks; others were offered on an ad hoc basis, that is,
agencies would ring up and suggest the child come to stay, while a few
parents had to rely on the goodwill of family members.

Extended family

Although not a formal service, breaks provided by families were part of the
patterns of care experienced by families, so are included here. Four of the

children had regular short breaks within their families, including two whose parents had separated. One ten-year-old boy had two married siblings who regularly took turns having him for a weekend, while a nine-year-old girl went to stay with her grandmother once a week. All the children seemed to accept these visits as part and parcel of their lives. In some cases it was viewed as a treat to be able to spend time with an older sister or favourite grandmother. It is noticeable, however, that for all the close contact between the children and their extended families, short breaks within the family happened in few cases. This may be another indication of the unease with which some extended family members viewed a disabled child and the lack of support they were consequently able to offer.

Voluntary organisations

Four children had short breaks in facilities run by voluntary organisations. For one girl these were regular and planned, for two boys they were occasional and usually at the suggestion of the organisation and for another girl, they were infrequent – mainly because she was reluctant to attend a residential facility. In two cases, the idea of a short break had been introduced to the child gradually: s/he was invited to see round the residence, stay for tea and chat to the other children before deciding whether or not to attend. One girl had an outreach worker from the facility who made regular contact with her family. This unit also had a procedure for involving children in aspects of service delivery, the only example reported in the study. For example, one 14-year-old boy had been involved in the appointment of new care staff:

> Child: The assistant manager left and we interviewed, we were interviewing all the different people, like the kids were interviewing them to find out what they were like.
>
> Interviewer: Uhuh. And what kinds of things did you ask?

Child: If they had any experience with disabled people. If they've ever lifted them and that and what would they do if somebody wanted to have fun but it was dangerous and can they take a joke...

The girl who attended this facility reported that she was very happy going to her 'hotel' while the boy, who did say he enjoyed himself, would have liked more outings. He did not like 'having to stay in and be bored'.

Another older girl in the sample had short breaks in a hospice, because there were no suitable placements in her locality. Initially, her whole family was invited to stay for the weekend but now she went on her own. She said she enjoyed her time at the hospice very much and was happy to keep going back. Her mother, however, had reservations about her daughter, whose condition was not immediately life threatening, staying in a place where, the mother felt, death was so evident:

> All the mums in the wee smoke room off loaded onto me about funerals and choosing coffins and things so with a lot of their kids it was imminent but with (Helen's condition) it's in the future, you want them to live and the hospice is, it's...it's...death's part of it, it's a natural part of it. Helen's got a lot of living to do, it's not the place for her. There should be a place that's respite for Helen and children with her disability.

Hospitals

Both the children with complex support needs had regular planned stays in the children's ward of a local hospital. One had previously gone to a social care facility but, after sustaining an injury there, was placed in hospital instead. One mother had put particular effort into educating hospital staff about her daughter's needs and had seen some improvement in her management. The parents of both children felt that short breaks on a hospital ward were not ideal: admitting children to medical settings for social reasons is generally recognised as poor practice. However, this was the only break on offer so each family felt they had to take it. Three issues troubled them. First, their already vulnerable children were being exposed to further infections on the ward and often returned home in poor health. Second, hospital staff were confused about the boundaries between an admission for medical reasons and a short break which happened to take place in a hospital. One child had all her medication changed during one admission: she was treated as a patient, not as a child having a break. Third, it was important but not always easy to ensure that the same nurses, who were familiar with the children's care plans, were with them through-out their stay. These nurses had worked with the children over a period of time and were well known to them. If any of these nurses was ill, the children's break was cancelled.

One of the young women, using non-verbal communication, fre-quently expressed her dislike of being away from her family. When asked how her daughter's short break could be managed better, her mother offered this suggestion:

> You could give Rhona the opportunity to do something in the time that she's not with us that is as enjoyable as what we would do when she's away. So it becomes a mutually beneficial experience for both of us…you will not think about placing children in a hospital or adults in a hospital. You will allow them the opportunity to do something that is typical, either home-based, if that's what the young person needs, or in the com-munity, or somewhere else that's fun, with ordinary people. It doesn't really take a lot.

Local authority placements

Two children had a mixture of short breaks. They were involved with 'be-friending' schemes: one boy had contact with an adult for a few hours each week, allowing his parents time with their other children; the boy who was at residential school had a befriender at home during school holidays. His mother had specifically requested that this adult help him learn about his local community. Both boys had further short breaks at regular intervals in local authority residential homes. Children and parents expressed neither like nor dislike of these placements.

Taken overall, the short breaks offered to disabled children and their families were very diverse in their duration, location and management. There was a feeling among parents of having to 'make do' with what was offered because they either accepted that or got nothing. In order to meet other needs, notably those of their other children, they felt forced to com-promise on what they wanted for their disabled child. There was a sense, too, of children having to fit into whatever facility was on offer, rather than creating a package to meet what each child needed. Only one child in the sample had regular, planned short breaks in a place which offered support to her, advice to her parents and an outreach worker whenever the need arose. Robinson (1996) suggests a number of other ways to manage short breaks. These will be discussed in Chapter 8.

Summary

Children were mostly positive about the professionals they encountered, albeit occasionally unclear about the difference between them. Parents' opinions were more qualified. They were enthusiastic about support received from voluntary organisations, reported helpful and unhelpful experiences with health professionals and felt they had to battle with some education professionals. Most families had little or no contact with social workers. Half the children had short breaks from their families. These took a variety of forms, ranging from the very ordinary experience of staying with extended family to the very atypical experience of being admitted to hospital for social reasons. Although there were exceptions, parents and children were rarely satisfied with the short breaks on offer.

Impairment effects are again evident in this chapter, the most obvious perhaps being the high level of health problems and need for medical treatment among the children. This was sometimes handled sensitively by professionals, but a lack of appropriate facilities had disabling effects in some cases. Other forms of discrimination encountered by some, but not all, of the children included a lack of suitable aids and equipment to support them in everyday activities, and 'inclusion' policies in school which were not enforced and in some cases actually served to exclude the child. While some professionals were good at involving children, in other cases failure to consult, or treating the young people in a childish way, can be seen as attacks on 'being' (Thomas 1999). Again there is evidence in these findings that those around the disabled child, in this case the parents, may also experience critical or unhelpful attitudes which impact adversely on their psycho-emotional well-being.

Chapter Six

Brothers and Sisters

Introduction

This chapter draws on interviews with 24 siblings of the disabled children and begins by describing their characteristics. It goes on to discuss roles and relationships, perceptions of difference, the reported effects of having a disabled brother or sister, siblings' worries and, finally, information provision and support.

Between them, the 26 disabled children had 40 brothers and sisters (four were only children). Siblings aged seven or older and living in the family home were sent an information sheet and agreement form, inviting them to take part in the research (see Appendices C and D). Four siblings declined to be interviewed and a fifth was not included at the request of his disabled brother and their mother: it was felt that the non-disabled boy was somewhat dominant, and it would be good for the disabled child to be the focus of some 'special' attention. Where there was more than one sibling, they had the choice of meeting the researcher separately or together. Eighteen interviews took place in all, including six with two children.

The children were asked about the time they spent with the disabled child and what they did together. They were asked how they would describe their brother or sister, how they got on together and what information they had been given about the sibling's impairment. They were asked what it was like having, for example, 'Jenny' as a sister, and follow-up prompts were used to explore good aspects and any 'not so good' aspects. The brothers and sisters were also asked if they thought having a disabled sibling was any different from having a non-disabled one, and if so, in what way. They were also asked about social work support and siblings' groups. There were two different versions of the interview guide, for older and younger children (see Appendix J).

Characteristics of the sample

The 24 siblings came from 14 families. There were 15 girls and 9 boys, aged between 6 and 19. (Two six-year-olds were included at their parents' request.) Four seven-year-olds also participated. The largest cluster was of children aged between 11 and 13, of whom there were ten. Fourteen siblings were older than the disabled child, eight were younger and two were twins of the disabled child. The total number of children in these families ranged from two to five. Two siblings were said by their parents to have an impairment themselves. One older brother had diagnoses of dyslexia and attention deficit hyperactivity disorder while one twin was currently being assessed for learning difficulties.

Roles and relationships

Positive aspects

Most children described their relationships with their disabled brother or sister in predominantly positive terms. There were three exceptions, to be discussed later. Many children spoke of their siblings with affection:

> It's good. I love her. She loves me.

> We are friends. She's always pleased to see me.

> He gets along with his big brother. He likes me baby-sitting.

> She's one of the best sisters I could ever have asked for.

Fourteen younger children were asked to complete a 'word choice' exercise, selecting words that described their disabled sibling. From the range of words offered:

- 'happy' and 'kind' were each selected by 12 children

- 'loving', 'clever', 'moody' and 'funny' (in the sense of telling funny jokes or making funny faces) were each selected by 11 children

- 'stubborn' was selected by 10 children

- 'annoying' and 'sad' were each selected by 9 children

- 'sleepy', 'helpful' and 'naughty' were each selected by 8 children

- 'hyper', 'embarrassing', 'different' and 'cool' were each selected by 7 children

- 'lazy' was selected by 5 children

- 'odd' was selected by 2 children.

Thus, siblings chose a mixture of 'positive' and 'negative' words, but five of the six selected most frequently were positive. Among the children seen as 'clever' were several with learning disabilities or communication difficulties. Where children were described as 'sad', 'different' or 'odd', these descriptors were not always related to the child's impairment, but attributed to some other aspect of her/his experience, or a response to a particular incident. These findings are very similar to those of Mackaskill (1985) who first used this type of exercise with siblings of adopted disabled children. She reports that 'quick' and 'clever' were often chosen, but 'odd' and 'different' were seldom selected.

The frequency with which words like 'helpful', 'loving' and 'kind' were selected indicates the potential for positive reciprocal relationships between disabled children and their siblings. The help given by the former and reported by the latter ranged from household chores to homework including, in two cases, helping an older non-disabled child with maths. One of the siblings getting this sort of help commented: 'She's a bit more clever than me.' The twin sister of a young girl with high support needs reported that the latter helped her in 'lots of ways' but did not specify what these were. In this case, it is possible that the child was referring to the closeness and affection which she felt towards her twin and which she believed was reciprocated. One girl with an autistic brother commented: 'If you are sad, he will come and give you a cuddle.'

Siblings' choice of words challenges some stereotypical views of people with certain impairments, for example that children with learning difficulties are 'stupid', or that those with autism are unempathic. Although this may not have been a conscious or deliberate action on the part of siblings, nevertheless, their choice to perceive their disabled brother or sister in these ways is evidence of agency on their part.

Activities and pastimes

There were many reports of shared activities and pastimes. Younger children, not surprisingly, spent time playing together – hide and seek and piggy-back apparently being favourites. Going out on their bikes, on family excursions, playing together with other local children or with cousins, and watching television and videos were all mentioned. Two young girls, whose brother was autistic and had no speech, played physical games with him, 'tried to interest him' in the computer and had developed one or two non-verbal signs to help him communicate with them.

Some older siblings also played with younger disabled children but were more likely to help them in various ways or help their parents look after them. However, this assistance usually took the form of 'a helping hand when needed' rather than frequent or substantial help. Two young people were more heavily involved in looking after their disabled sibling, as will be discussed later.

Although most children did not play a significant role in looking after their siblings in a practical sense, several expressed some sense of responsibility for the disabled child. Most were aware that their sibling was less able or more vulnerable than them in some respects and several of the non-disabled children expressed protective feelings towards their sibling.

A few children did not spend much time with their disabled sibling. This included two brothers whose sister had complex support needs and limited ability to communicate. While they were fond of her, and anxious about her well-being, they reported that they did not see a great deal of her, especially during week-days. This girl, whose health required constant monitoring, appeared to spend a good deal of time in her own room, with a parent or nurse in attendance. There was a sense in which the boys and their sister lived parallel lives.

Ups and downs

Those who did generally get on well with their disabled brother or sister nevertheless reported having 'fights' or arguments at times. With younger children, this often took the form of bickering over who owned a particular toy, or what game to play; with older children, there were disagreements about what television programme to watch. One six-year-old said: '(He) can be quite good fun to play with, he can be rubbish.' Similarly, an 11-year-old said of his younger sister: 'We get on okay if she gives me space... She's annoying and nice.' The sisters of the autistic boy mentioned above, while clearly very fond of him, admitted that he could be annoying at times, tearing up paper and colouring or scribbling on their books. However, they had 'more fun than fights'.

The 'ups and downs' described by these children seem very typical of sibling relationships generally. One mother said of her children: 'They get on like two normal siblings.' Three siblings compared the disabled child favourably to another sibling. For example, one seven-year-old described her 13-year-old non-disabled sister as always 'bossy' and 'busy' whereas her ten-year-old disabled sister was 'kind, fun and helpful'. One ten-year-old described how he and his disabled twin sometimes 'ganged up' on their 'annoying' little sister.

Problematic aspects

A few children who presented their relationships in predominantly positive terms nevertheless clearly had ambivalent feelings towards their sibling, to a more marked degree than the ups and downs described above. The most striking of these was Tracey, a 19-year-old woman who reported fighting with her 16-year-old brother 'like cat and dog'. On occasion he would attack Tracey, leaving her with visible bruising and scratches. Over the years, other people's reactions to her brother had led to a number of unpleasant experiences for Tracey. She had been badly bullied at school, had lost boyfriends and her current social life was severely restricted by having to sit with her brother at weekends while their single mother went out to work. Tracey added that at one point she had felt she hated her brother, and that this in turn had made her hate herself. At the same time, she expressed great affection for him – 'I love him to pieces' – and reported her intention that he should live with her when their mother was no longer able to care for him. The ambivalence apparent in her account seems to reflect a dichotomy between her genuine feelings of affection for her brother and her resentment of the negative impact on her own life.

Thomas (1999) did not extend her thesis about a 'social relational' understanding of disability, encompassing the idea of restrictions on being and doing, to people around the disabled individual. However, our findings raise questions about whether the experiences and restrictions faced by some parents and siblings could have a place in that model or, perhaps more likely, can be better understood through that model. We have already noted indications that parents of disabled children, although without an impairment themselves, may be affected by attacks on their psycho-emotional well-being through the offensive remarks of relatives, or the insensitive behaviour of professionals.

Tracey's experience suggests that brothers and sisters of disabled children can also experience attacks on their psycho-emotional well-being which, in Tracey's case, left her feeling unhappy and angry. She also experienced restrictions of activity, in the sense that her social life was curtailed while she sat with her brother, although this was a temporary arrangement until she went to university later that year. These restrictions were not, of course, the 'result' of disability: they were caused by a combination of circumstances including her mother's single parent status and financial circumstances, and the lack of formal support particularly in the form of a sitting service. We will take up this theme again in Chapter 8.

As mentioned above, three children had poor relationships with their disabled siblings. This included a sibling pair, a boy aged 11 and a girl aged seven, whose nine-year-old brother was said to have a mild physical impairment and 'challenging behaviour'. There were two other children in this family who declined to be interviewed. The older boy made no positive comments about his brother, but described him as 'really bad', physically attacking the other children; they never had any fun together and did not like each other. The girl spoke in very similar terms, although she did say some more positive things when presented with the 'word circle.' It is hard to tell how much the disabled child did in fact initiate trouble, and how much he reacted to being provoked or excluded by the others, since he was said to attack them 'when some of us annoy him', and 'if some of us squirt him with water'. When the disabled boy was interviewed, he described his siblings attacking him for no apparent reason.

Finally, a 13-year-old boy had very little good to say about his nine-year-old sister, who had been diagnosed with a form of attention deficit hyperactivity disorder (ADHD). He said he could not think of anything he liked about her. The siblings spent little time together except when visiting their father at weekends. The boy found her behaviour embarrassing (for example, kissing his friends, then hitting him) and said he 'felt strange' about her. This boy also described his sister as arguing with him and physically attacking him for no reason: 'One day she was hitting, she was going mental at me, so she hit me with my belt right across my face.'

However, it is worth noting that this boy also had a recent diagnosis of ADHD, and began the interview by giving a graphic account of having attacked another boy at school, apparently quite violently. As in the case above, when the disabled child was interviewed, she also related how her brother lashed out at her for no apparent reason. Clearly these three relationships, which are qualitatively distinct from the rest of the sample, are linked by accounts of physical attacks. It is not surprising that siblings experience difficult relationships when this level of challenging behaviour is present in one or more of them. Three other young people had similar experiences but these did not appear to mar their relationships to the same extent. One of them was Tracey; in another case, the attack described appeared to be a one-off incident; the third was Jenny, a 12-year-old girl who said of her younger brother: 'He's a little bit naughty to me…sometimes kicks, punches, pushes me down the stairs.'

It was not clear what mitigating factors led Jenny to present the relationship with her brother in predominantly positive terms. It may be that her brother's attacks were less frequent or less severe than those perpetrated by other children, or that she had greater understanding of the reasons for his behaviour, allowing her to tolerate it better. However, Jenny later expressed anxiety about saying something which might upset her parents; it is possible that concern about articulating more negative feelings led her to censor some responses. We come back to this point later.

Perceptions of difference

Hames (1998) analysed the comments of 11 pre-school children about their disabled older siblings, and observed their interactions. She found that some of the infants copied their disabled sibling and wanted to be the same as them. Others wanted their older brother or sister to be like them (for example, able to walk or talk). Third, and this was more common as they grew older, some pre-school children copied their parents' behaviour towards the disabled child, mainly by helping her/him. Hames concludes that very young children start by seeing, or looking for, similarities but before long become aware of significant differences. Her study was, however, focused on developmental aspects of childhood. Smith and Williams (2001) explored the perceptions of children aged 4–12 who did not have disabled siblings and had little or no direct contact with children with impairments. Overall, these children had a positive perception of the capabilities of children with different types of impairment, although some age differences were found.

In this study, children were asked, at the beginning of the interview, how they would describe their disabled sibling to someone who had never met her/him. Most did not include any reference to impairment in their response. Younger children tended to describe the child in terms of his appearance: 'He's annoying; he's got ginger hair, he wears glasses and he's got loads of freckles. Err, he likes to climb trees.' Others described aspects of their sibling's personality, often emphasising that he or she was a happy child: 'He laughs a lot. And he makes fun of you a lot. And he can be good company sometimes…happy…most of the time.' Some children described their sibling more in terms of the relationship: 'Normally happy; I know she loves me; she smiles and laughs at me and looks at me.'

Some children were more explicit about the 'ordinariness' of their disabled brother or sister:

> She's just really like any other normal ten-year-old. I don't see her as being deaf. I just see her as a normal child.

> I mention his disability when I describe him, but that's not my focal point. I don't see him as a disability. I see him as Steven, so.

When asked if she had any friends with a sister 'like Mary', a seven-year-old replied: 'a twin sister?' Similarly, a five-year-old, asked if she knew any other children 'like her brother', replied that she did, and went on to describe her male cousin who was of a similar age and liked some similar activities. These findings coincide with those of Mackaskill (1985) and Lobato (1990) who found that most children did not include references to impairment when describing their disabled brother or sister. Again, in constructing these positive accounts of their siblings, there is evidence of agency on the part of these children. Two siblings did, however, refer to the child's impairment in their initial description of her: 'She's got a learning difficulty…it slows all her… She's different…like she cannie really do anything.'

Most children thought that having a disabled sister or brother was little different from having a non-disabled sibling. Several commented that the situation was 'normal' for them or that they had never known anything different. This included a few children who described their sibling, or the experience of having a disabled sibling, as 'different'. This did not usually carry a negative connotation:

> Because I've lived with him all my life, I don't see him as any different anyway.

> Even although she's deaf, I still play with her and she suits me fine.

> Well (having a non-disabled sister) wouldn't really change anything. I would still just have a sister and I would love her.

> She's different but it's normal for us.

Some children identified positive benefits from having a disabled sibling. One felt that her brother was 'not as nasty' as her friends' non-disabled brothers; another believed that, as a result of his experiences, his younger brother was more mature and philosophical than a non-disabled brother of the same age might be. Most children accepted the impairment as part of the sibling and did not see any reason to wish it changed: 'It wouldn't be the same if Carol wasn't here' and 'I couldn't have a life without annoyance!'

However, a few children thought that having a disabled sibling entailed more significant differences than those quoted above. In one case, the difference centred on the fact that the child's brother had a life-limiting illness. On the one hand, this girl described with great feeling her conviction that her brother's physical impairment did not alter his essential humanity:

> I don't mind John being in the wheelchair, like he is my brother and that's it. He is just usually like any other boys that walk about in the streets apart from the fact that John's legs don't work. That's the only thing that I see different. He's still a human with like still the same face and same body, but some people look at him as if he has got horns on his head.

At the same time, this girl was aware that her brother's condition did single him out from other children, since he was struggling to come to terms with a future very different from that facing his peers. She too would be happier if he could 'get on with his life' like other teenagers. A few younger children sometimes felt frustrated that their disabled sibling could not play certain games with them, help them with 'big sums', or had difficulty hearing them. One regretted that he could not talk to his sister about what was happening in his life.

Some siblings displayed considerable sensitivity when describing their disabled brother or sister, trying to imagine how it must feel to be 'different' or to have experiences which differed from the rest of the family or from 'the norm'. For example, one teenager wished he could understand more about how his younger brother felt about being moved to a special school, especially when his twin remained in mainstream education. A few children believed that their disabled siblings were over-sensitive at times, liable to interpret comments the wrong way, or to think that others were laughing at them. They attributed this heightened sensitivity to the fact that their brother or sister had an impairment. This made one girl rather cautious about what she said to her brother, and thought that he in turn viewed her as 'nicey nicey'. On the other hand, among those children with markedly poor relationships, there was a noticeable lack of empathy with the disabled child. One of these children said he could not understand why his sister behaved in the way she did; another was asked how he felt when his younger brother cried and banged his head on the wall. He replied: 'Nothing... I just ignore it and watch TV.' He believed his brother showed difficult behaviour because he was 'really bad'.

The effects of having a disabled sibling

Activities and going out

As explained at the start of this chapter, the young people were asked fairly general questions about having a disabled brother or sister, and to identify any good and less good aspects. The data presented below reflect the range of responses given: it should be borne in mind that the children were not specifically asked to comment on each of these domains.

It has been reported that the brothers and sisters of disabled children are greatly restricted in the range of activities they can pursue and that family outings may be virtually impossible (e.g. Widdows 1997). That was not the picture presented by most children in this study. Five made no reference to constraints on their activities while six stated that there were none. The latter group tended to be older children who could go out and about by themselves or with friends; two of them thought that their younger sibling was more restricted by having a disabled brother or sister than they were. Six children reported that there were some places they could not go with the disabled child. One reported that her family was not able to go abroad as often as they would like. Another teenager had a slightly different experience: he was increasingly fed-up with pressure from his mother to join the family at events run by organisations for disabled people, when he would rather be off with his own friends. Although his father sympathised with his feelings, the boy continued to attend these events (he said) through a sense of guilt.

Again, these are examples of non-disabled children having their activities restricted through a combination of circumstances. This is also well illustrated in the account of two brothers whose parents had decided that if a particular place or activity was not accessible to their disabled daughter, thus preventing the whole family doing something together, then none of them would do it. Thus, the brothers were not able to go to the funfair or the beach, and while on holiday had not been able to go to the harbour or to certain tourist attractions. In these scenarios, it could be argued that the children were adversely affected by the same barriers as their disabled sister. However, their parents responded differently from most others in this study, who sought to minimise the adverse impact of such barriers on their non-disabled children. In this case, the parents' efforts to avoid excluding the disabled child from family activity resulted in her brothers being excluded from ordinary, age appropriate activities. This example also illustrates the potentially ambiguous role of parents. In this instance, to what extent were they affected by the same barriers as the disabled child, a process identified by Rose (1997), or alternatively, how far did they contribute to or cause the problem by the way they chose to handle the situation?

One or two siblings were able to identify some bonuses in terms of activities. At Disneyland, for example, families received preferential treatment because of the disabled child. Other siblings identified compensations. For example, one family could not travel on public transport with the child, but they could ring Dial-A-Ride. Three children reported that their siblings went into short-term care to allow the family to have a break. Thus, although there were some restrictions most of the time, they did have a regular break when they could pursue activities of their own choice. However, these young people had ambivalent feelings about short-term care. In two cases the disabled child was having a 'break' in a hospital setting and the siblings were clearly doubtful about the appropriateness of this arrangement. Second, they worried that the child felt 'lonely' or 'left out'. Third, there was the uneasy feeling that this unsatisfactory arrangement had been made at least partly for their own benefit. One 12-year-old commented: 'I think it's better if she's not here 'cause we get to, like do a lot more things but sometimes I feel like she's a bit left out and I don't know what to do about that.' An eight-year-old said: 'But when I'm on holiday I worry a little about her at the hospital.'

Overall, however, the children reported what may seem, given previous findings elsewhere, relatively few restrictions on their activities as a result of having a disabled sibling. Those that were reported appeared to be accepted as part of everyday life. A few children added that their parents had tried to restrict any negative impact on their activities and to encourage them to have 'normal' lives.

Relationships with parents

Previous research has suggested that one of the main effects of having a disabled child in the family is that her/his siblings receive less time and attention from their parents, sometimes with further damaging consequences (Meltzer *et al.* 1989). Again, this was not borne out by the majority of our respondents, 18 of whom made no mention of feeling they had 'lost out' in this way. Four siblings reported that they saw less of their parents than they might otherwise have done. For example, a 14-year-old boy said:

> It's just sometimes I'd like to come in and talk about something, but they're tied up or they're going out or something... I'm not saying anything bad about Florence, but if she wasn't disabled then my mum wouldn't have got involved with all these groups and everything and then she'd just be at work, and then she'd have more time for me and Paula [his non-disabled sister] and Florence.

The three other children who reported they saw less of their parents because of the disabled child also stated that this did not 'bother' them. Two of these were older teenagers who were perhaps relatively independent of their parents, and whose disabled sibling was a good deal younger. However, Jenny, the girl who was worried about upsetting her parents, admitted that her brother got his own way too much and that this was not really fair. She later had this exchange with the interviewer:

Jenny:	If I want to do something with my mum and George's not feeling well or George needs something, then Mum can't do it with me.
Interviewer:	Right, uhuh. So do you ever feel kind of left out?
Jenny:	No.
Interviewer:	No. And it's okay that George has to come first, is it?
Jenny:	Uhuh.

Interviewer: Uhuh. And do you ever feel angry about it?

Jenny: No.

Interviewer: No. Or feel sad?

Jenny: No.

Jenny was not the only child who was protective towards her parents, and this is not the first study to find that siblings try to shield their parents from further worries by keeping things to themselves (see Tozer 1996).

Siblings' friendships

Few of the children reported that having a disabled sibling had any impact on their own friendships. Most said their friends knew their sibling and in many cases got on well together. One teenager said of his younger brother: 'He's got a cheeky side to him which a lot of my pals find quite funny, him being the age he is – the wee guy who hings aboot them a'. He's a nice person.'

There were some reports, particularly where brothers and sisters were closer in age, of friends coming to visit siblings and ending up spending more time with the disabled child. The young people did not say they minded or were jealous about this, although that might have been a natural reaction, especially among younger children. A couple of siblings commented that their friends did not understand what it was like to have a disabled brother or sister; they did not indicate that their friends were uncaring but simply that they lacked the same experience. This could make it difficult for children to discuss their feelings about having a disabled sibling with their friends. Two children actively avoided discussing the subject with their friends, in one case, on his mother's instructions: 'I just want to keep it between…my mum said just keep it in between our family.' Another child, who tried to change the subject if friends he brought home asked questions about his sister, did so because he had been taunted at school.

As already noted, 19-year-old Tracey had experienced considerable difficulty in terms of impact on relationships. She had lost a number of boyfriends who apparently could not cope with the fact that she had a disabled brother. Hurtful remarks had been made to her on this subject: 'I had one serious boyfriend who thought…he sort of looked at me and went, "If you ever have kids they're going to be like this". Said it to my face and walked out as well.' Although clearly upset at the time, Tracey had since rationalised the situation to the effect that anyone with this attitude was not a desirable partner anyway.

Bullying and taunting

Five siblings had experienced taunting or bullying at school about having a disabled brother or sister, in some cases for prolonged periods:

> It was very difficult trying to explain it all to my peers, and I got bullied for a while at school… I mean a lot of times it was, 'Your brother's thick, it means you're thick'. Bla, bla, bla. I don't like when people that are not my friends say, 'You've got a stupid sister, I've got a better sister', like that.

Not surprisingly, these children had been upset and angered by the way they had been treated, again suggesting that they too could experience 're-strictions on being' (Thomas 1999). At the same time, their responses in dealing with bullying indicates active agency. Two had never told their parents about the problem – 'I just try to hide it from everyone', said one. 'I just keep it to myself' said another. In addition, one commented that teachers were unaware of the bullying. Another child mentioned that when she had given a talk to her class about her brother and the condition he had, it was the first time her teacher realised she had a disabled sibling.

Demands on siblings to help

Beresford (1994) reports that young siblings do not generally carry out 'unusual' care tasks but do what any child might do to help a brother or sister. Most children in this study did not play a significant role in looking after their disabled sibling. Where they did help out, this was often on a 'voluntary' basis and consisted of the kind of assistance that older children might offer younger siblings in any family, such as helping them get dressed, organised for school or keeping an eye on them when their parents were otherwise occupied. The difference in some cases was that the disabled child was of an age when such help would not usually be required, or was older than the helping sibling. Two brothers had been shown how to lift their sister onto the toilet or into her wheelchair 'in a special way, so that it willna' hurt her'. Three young people reported that they looked after their disabled siblings when their parents were out, but this appeared to be on an occasional basis and not for long periods. Again there was a sense that many parents did not wish to make demands on their non-disabled children, nor disrupt their normal activities. Looking after the disabled child was seen as primarily a parental responsibility. Only two girls reported providing regular help. One was Tracey, whose mother seemed to expect her to do so. The other was a 12-year-old, who 'fetched and carried' for her older brother after school. This was not expected by her parents, who employed a child-minder, and the girl resented what she saw as her brother's demanding attitude.

Other effects

Several children stated that having a disabled sibling had little overall impact and had not affected the way they had been brought up. Others did identify additional effects besides those discussed above. Five children, all of whose disabled siblings had been bullied or taunted, usually by children but sometimes by adults, believed they were more aware and accepting of difference than they would otherwise have been. Some had a strong sense of injustice about the way their sibling was treated by others. A 13-year-old, whose future ambition was to help children with disabled siblings 'sort out their feelings', commented: 'Then say Robert wasn't here… I'd probably react differently to people that had a disability than I do now… I just find it really hard to cope with people that don't under- stand and are really horrible about it…'

A few children had defended their siblings from name calling and derogatory remarks made by others:

> Sometimes it's really annoying if someone will look at him, as if 'What are you?' 'That's my brother you are looking at.' I said that to somebody and they were standing watching my brother and she just stood and looked at him. And I said, 'What are you looking at?' She looked at me and walked away and tons of wee, not wee, like girls about the same age as me, all come round and look at him and I just go like that and put my

> hand on my hips and they will just turn away... Sometimes folk just stare at him and it must make him feel like dirt.

Tracey believed that being bullied at school, although clearly an unhappy experience, had made her a stronger person. She also felt that looking after her brother had made her more responsible and mature than she might otherwise have been.

Two sibling pairs felt they received less attention from other people – besides their parents – than did their disabled sibling. One of these children saw her sister as the 'teacher's pet' and felt this was unfair. Another reported that family, friends and relations always asked after the disabled child first and generally paid greater attention to her than to the two non-disabled children. While able to rationalise this, there remained a lingering sense of injustice.

Worries about the child

The children were asked if they ever worried about their disabled sibling. Nearly all of them did. In a few cases, children seemed to have a high level of on-going anxiety about the child's well-being. One such boy, aged 12, said of his sister:

> When we were at St Andrews, it was the first time with the...new wheel-chair, and my mum had went down a step and the wheelchair had tipped, and that night I had had a dream that we were all on this hill beside the seaside, and Cathy had took off her brakes and she had went rolling into the sea.

The subject of most concern was the child's health and physical well-being. Three children were worried about their sibling's prognosis; a few were anxious when the child went into hospital for operations or treatment, and some were concerned that the child was prone to accidents. The other main cause of concern focused on people bullying the child or taking advantage of her/him in some way. In some cases, this fear stemmed from real experience of the child being ill-treated; in others, the concern was more about potential vulnerability. As previously noted, three children were concerned that their sibling felt lonely or left out while in short-term care.

Other worries, each of which was mentioned by only one or two siblings, included:

- seeing their parents distressed about the disabled child
- worry that the child could not play alongside other (non-disabled) children
- concern about a sister who sometimes 'wandered off' for long periods
- a more generalised sense of responsibility and concern for a child's well-being
- the possibility that the sibling might have disabled children herself.

Support for siblings

Information and opportunities for discussion

While some children could discuss their worries with either or both parents, this was not true for all. Indeed, there is cause for concern that a few children had apparently been told little or nothing about their sibling's condition. Others, who had been given some information, nevertheless felt they had not been told much, or as much as they wanted to know. One girl, who was five when her sister's impairment was diagnosed, commented:

> Maybe if my mum and dad had tried to explain to me what was going on, but they didn't, they just, I'm not saying anything bad about them but...I'd see them really upset and crying and I'd want to know what was wrong but they'd just say 'Oh, it was nothing'. So I think, if there was someone else going through it now, I think their parents should try and explain what was happening because my mum and dad never did that with me.

Several children said that, although they would like more opportunity to discuss the implications of their sibling's condition or to talk about how they felt about having a disabled brother or sister, they did not wish to raise these subjects with their parents. Usually this seemed to be a means of protecting their parents, some of whom apparently became upset if asked the 'wrong' questions. Jenny would have liked to find out more about her brother's condition:

Interviewer: Could you ask Mum and Dad again?

Jenny: Maybe.

Interviewer: But you aren't keen.

Jenny: No.

Interviewer: Why not?

Jenny: Don't know. Just too scared to ask.

Interviewer: Are you?

Jenny: Uhuh.

Interviewer: Why is it a bit scary?

Jenny: Just don't want to ask just in case I say something that my mum and dad wouldn't like me saying.

In one or two cases, however, there were hints of a stigma being associated with the presence of impairment within the family, as in the case of the boy whose mother had told him 'to keep it in between the family'. This teenager had gone to the library and surfed the Internet to find out more information about his sister's condition, rather than ask his parents.

Two young people wanted to talk to their disabled sibling more openly but either sensed that the latter did not wish to do so or found it difficult themselves. This included a boy with a life-limiting condition whose sister said:

> He'll drop the odd comment, like the other night he says something about dying and I told him to shut up, and he says 'Do you not want to talk about it?' And I say 'No' 'cos I don't like talking but I don't try and change the subject, 'cos I know he is going through it as well...

A few children had talked about having a disabled sibling to someone outside the immediate family. These listeners were a mix of informal and professional contacts. Four commented that the research interview was the first time they had ever spoken to anyone outside the family. One teenager, when visiting her brother's special school, had noticed 'a few of the kids, (i.e. siblings), people like my age, standing there looking totally bewildered'. She felt that much more should be done to inform and support siblings.

Siblings' groups

Eight young people, including three sibling pairs, had attended groups or events for siblings of disabled children. There were mixed views about these groups. One pair attended siblings' activities run by a voluntary organisation every weekend, the younger one having a choice of arts and crafts, sports and games and a soft play area, while the teenager attended a discussion group. She found it helpful to talk to other people 'with the same problems' and could ring up other group members at home if she felt in need of support. Another forum which worked well for one girl was a siblings' weekend run in a children's hospice; again, the opportunity to talk to other children with disabled siblings was appreciated. She also commented:

> I have been feeling it a lot easier because the person that is with me then is like my own age, and like the words we use some adults don't understand…it's usually the people that are over 23 that don't understand.

Two brothers were attending a young carers' group held every week at a voluntary agency. A meal and various recreational activities were provided and occasional weekend trips organised. They enjoyed these sessions, which appeared to be purely social, giving siblings the chance to have 'a break' (as their parents put it) and pursue activities they might not manage as a family. There was no formal discussion about having a disabled brother or sister, although the boys had been asked by other siblings 'who we're here for'.

However, other children had found siblings' groups less satisfactory. One boy had been upset by going to a siblings' event at the children's hospice because he had seen other children, with the same condition as his sister, whose illness was more advanced. Another child, who had been the youngest in her group, felt left out and eventually stopped going. Two sisters attending a group elsewhere had not gained much from the experience, again partly due to being a different age from other members.

However, the older sister had talked to one boy there and had found that helpful, since her own friends 'don't know what it feels like'.

Among children who had never been to a siblings' group, only three said they would like to try going: others were not attracted to the idea or did not know if they would like it or not. Several children would have liked to talk to someone outside the family about some aspect of having a disabled sibling but were not sure whom. There was not a lot of enthusiasm for talking to professionals, and there was some concern that anything they said should remain confidential; this again was related to anxiety about upsetting parents.

Comparison with parents' views

Overall, the young people's accounts of their relationships with their disabled brothers and sisters, and of the impact on family life, were similar to those of their parents. Most parents described their children's relationships in very ordinary terms: several referred to them as 'normal' siblings. For example, a teenage girl who had described 'holding back' from her brother who had a poor prognosis, was described by her mother as 'distancing herself... We almost became two families in here.' Tracey's mother said she argued with her brother 'like normal siblings' but 'adored' him. One seven-year-old had described a very ordinary relationship with her nine-year-old brother. Her mother wryly commented: 'She cannot control her indifference at times.' The parents of the 13-year-old boy who did not like his sister described the siblings' relationship in ways which closely matched the boy's account: 'That's a non-existence. (He) don't want to know. That's an open time bomb.'

Echoing the tenor of what some siblings had said, several parents reported they had made conscious efforts over the years to ensure their non-disabled children were not adversely affected by having a disabled child in the family. However, several acknowledged that the disabled child had received more time and attention than her/his brothers and sisters and a few thought that the latter felt some jealousy and resentment about this. Indeed, parents were more likely than their children to report jealous or resentful feelings. Whether this was because parents imagined their non-disabled children felt these emotions more than they actually did (perhaps because parents felt guilty about not spending more time with their non-disabled sons and daughters), or whether siblings did harbour such feelings but were reluctant to mention them, is unclear.

In contrast to some children's accounts of limited communication with parents about their disabled sibling, most parents reported they had discussed the subject openly. It is possible that the disparity in perceptions is due to some parents not realising that their children wanted more information, or more opportunity to talk and ask questions. A couple of parents were aware that their non-disabled children were trying to protect them. Shelley (1998) has suggested that parents may also want to protect their non-disabled children from unnecessary pain and from feeling 'burdened'. For this reason, parents may ration or censor the information they pass on.

Most parents reported that little support, particularly of a formal nature, was available to siblings. One mother commented:

> We never discussed it in her presence but obviously she overheard a lot, and I can't quite remember what age she was. She was quite, she was maybe seven or eight and we discovered she was telling people things, talking to people, and then we had to be more open, especially me, her father was quite, em, uncommunicative about it. But no, she's had no support. Only from me, and I'm normally no good.

Another parent said: 'We've done it ourselves 'cos there's not a lot of support groups. There's Alteen and the ones for gamblers and Cruise but there's nothing for the likes of Muriel and Hannah...'

Summary

Interviews were held with 24 brothers and sisters of the disabled children, aged 6 to 19. Their accounts were predominantly positive, often challenging stereotypes of disabled children and their potential for reciprocal relationships. The children who generally got on well together still had their disagreements but, for the most part, these ups and downs seemed to fall well within the 'normal' range of sibling relationships. However, there were a few significant exceptions, including some acrimonious and even violent relationships.

Siblings varied in the extent to which they saw the disabled child as 'different'. There was a strong sense of everyday life being 'ordinary' – or ordinary for them. Overall, siblings did not report that having a disabled child in the family had significant effects on their own lives, although there was evidence of restriction on the activities undertaken by some younger children. Five siblings had experienced bullying and taunting, usually at school.

However, a few children admitted they were careful not to 'bother' their parents with requests for time, attention or even information about their sibling's condition. Two never told their parents they had been bullied, while a couple who did report some restrictions on their lives stressed they were not blaming the disabled child. Thus, it is difficult to avoid speculating to what extent some children may have understated the impact of having a disabled sibling. Similarly, in a few cases, it is difficult to draw clear conclusions about how far their experiences helped the children become more mature and self-sufficient individuals, and how far they were left struggling to resolve difficult issues without support.

A few children were quite clear about negative effects. One young girl felt she had lost out in terms of the time and attention she received from her parents and another found her current social life greatly restricted by having to take on responsibility for her brother. Most of the children worried about their disabled siblings, particularly about their health and physical well-being. Many did not think they had been given sufficient information about the child's impairment or prognosis. Eight had been to siblings' groups; while some children found these helpful, others did not. Overall, little formal support was available for siblings.

Finally, at various points in this chapter it has been suggested that brothers and sisters are vulnerable to attacks on their psycho-emotional well-being. Some also experienced restrictions of activity, caused by a combination of factors and rather different from the barriers to 'doing' experienced by disabled children. However, it could also be argued that, in a small minority of cases, siblings themselves placed restrictions on disabled children's psycho-emotional well-being, through hurtful remarks and, occasionally, violent behaviour. Similarly, the potential for parents to impose restrictions on their non-disabled children was noted.

Chapter Seven

Children's Understandings of Disability

Introduction

Thomas's (1999) work has already been used to help illustrate the difference between an impairment, which in Western culture can be understood as a variation in the structure, function and working of the body, and disability: '...a form of social oppression involving the social imposition of restrictions of activity on people with impairments and the socially engendered undermining of their psycho-emotional well-being' (p.156).

To recap briefly, disability is rooted in an unequal social relationship, the effects of which can manifest themselves as barriers – physical, social and emotional – restricting the lives of disabled people. Thomas distinguishes between restrictions of activity (or barriers to 'doing') which result from disability, and psycho-emotional disablism (or barriers to 'being') such as being stared at, laughed at or made to feel unattractive – all of which impinge on an individual's self worth. She further distinguishes these manifestations of disability from the experience of living with impairment and impairment effects. Drawing on her framework, this chapter examines how far and in what ways disabled children perceive, and try to make sense of, difference and inequalities in their lives and the barriers which result from these inequalities. It also looks at the way their siblings perceive and understand impairment and disability.

Disabled children's understandings of disability

Perceptions of impairment

Disabled children were not asked directly how they understood disability: much of the detail in this section has been inferred from their accounts, with additional material from parents. Much of what the children named as disability was, in fact, about their 'impairment' and its effects, notably the medical and health implications, on their lives. The word impairment was not used by any of the children, suggesting that information about the social model of disability was not reaching them. So, the starting point for this section is an overview of how the disabled children understood impairment and where their information about it came from.

The main source of information, not surprisingly, seemed to be their parents. Many parents described feelings of dread when their child had asked why he or she had an impairment. It was not a topic which most parents discussed regularly with their child, rather, it seemed the child had asked once, often at quite a young age, after which the subject was not raised again. However, there was evidence of more discussion taking place with children whose conditions were deteriorating and therefore subject to change. Parental explanations usually focused on one or a mixture of the following: the cause of the impairment, the role of God or God's will, and the 'specialness' of the child.

Causes of the impairment were dealt with in terms of a mother's illness or an accident at birth. There did not seem to be any attempt to blame anyone for the child's impairment nor was there any evidence of it being viewed in a 'tragic' way. The mother of a 13-year-old girl answered her daughter's question about the cause of impairment thus:

> It was along these lines, that she was very special and that God had picked us to look after her and her to look after us as well. And she was quite happy with that. She just went, 'Oh right, okay' and that was it and she's never asked again.

One parent refused to think of her child in those terms:

> I sit and read these things about people saying 'Oh he's given me so much; he's so special and he's a gift from God.' That's a lot of shit. If I could have had three healthy, able-bodied children, I'd have them...

Some parents tried to protect their child from too much knowledge about the worst outcomes of any medical condition, although one mother reported that her daughter went through phases of talking about her death. This mother described how the girl had learned that her condition was life-limiting through gossip at school:

> We were just sitting and Rosemary said, 'You know, it's all round school that I'm going to die. Is that true?' And we sat and talked about it and I had to be honest. It was the hardest thing I've had to do in my life.

A number of the children did not and had not talked about their impairment to their parents. It may be that, for them, the presence of impairment in their lives was not of great significance. When disabled children were asked if there was anything in their lives they would like to change, only two referred to their impairment, saying they would like to be able to walk. Some young people with sensory and physical impairments were then asked a direct question about having their impairment removed; one boy would have preferred to have better vision and the rest declared themselves content to be the way they were. An older girl compared herself to some of her friends and felt she came off best: 'When I see people as they two are I think, "Gosh" and I'm like glad I can walk and people see me and I walk like this and they say, "Great, she can do that and we can't".'

A younger girl, with a hearing impairment, did not want to change anything about herself. This reflects a conversation which took place with her sisters about having 'three wishes', reported by her mother:

> And Julie was last and I was dreading what Julie would say. I thought she might say she wished she wasn't deaf but she didn't mention it...and later on when it was just Julie and I, I said to her, 'Do you wish that you weren't deaf?' and she said, 'No'. And I said, 'Why is that?' and she said, 'Because I wouldn't know or have all the special friends that I've got.' And I thought that was a lovely thing to say.

When one of the younger boys was asked if he ever wished he did not have to use a wheelchair, he gave a practical reply: 'That's it, I'm in a wheelchair so just get on with it. Just get on with what you're doing.'

Thus, the majority of the children interviewed seemed to be happy with themselves and not looking for a 'cure'. Impairment was never viewed in terms of a tragedy, rather, those children who mentioned it seemed very 'matter of fact' about it. The children had much more to say about the medical facets of their impairment than about the impairment itself. They described surgical procedures, hospital stays and visits, physiotherapy and decisions about future surgery. The children's focus on medical aspects of impairment suggests that, for most of them, impairment was seen primarily in medical terms. This is not surprising, given that most had high levels of contact with health professionals and little opportunity for contact with anyone who would challenge such a view. At the same time, the 'medical' model of disability and the 'personal tragedy' model are often equated: it is interesting and important that the children seemed to separate them. None of the children referred to feelings of loss or a sense that they had been 'hard done by'. Instead, they seemed to adopt a very practical, pragmatic approach.

At the same time, it is possible that some of the younger children may have thought they would 'outgrow' their impairment. When asked what they would do when they grew up, and whether they would need any help, only one of the younger children said that she would. It is not clear why the others felt they would not require help as adults. It may be that, as a number of them said, they expected to be still living at home with their parents. However, the mother of a nine-year-old boy with a hearing impairment reported that her son had gone through a 'phase' of believing that he would grow up into a hearing adult. She felt this belief came from not having any contact with deaf adults: all the adults in his world were hearing so he assumed that, one day, he would be too. Indeed, none of the other younger children seemed to have contact with disabled adults. In contrast, the older children were more likely to recognise they would need support to lead their adult lives and, again, adopted a pragmatic attitude towards it.

Other children described 'impairment effects' – the restrictions of 'doing' and 'being' which result from living with an impairment. For example, some of the children talked about the effects of impairment on their health. A 14-year-old boy wanted to live abroad so that he could avoid the detrimental effects of winter; he had repeated chest infections because of his condition and was regularly hospitalised to manage them. One girl described the pain that her impairment sometimes caused her.

Thomas (1999) stresses the importance of separating these 'impairment effects' from restrictions imposed on disabled people as a result of living in an unequal relationship with the rest of society. The children described a range of other experiences – restrictions of 'being' and 'doing' related to disability, not impairment – which did indeed seem to give them information about being in an unequal relationship. These are discussed in the following sections.

Barriers to 'being'
THE MANAGEMENT OF DIFFERENCE

On occasions, disabled children came up against situations which illustrated their difference from their peers. Parents thought that children were usually aware of themselves as different, although the children did not mention it; their focus was on the 'sameness' of their lives rather than the difference. This is interesting in that it must have been difficult for the children to avoid or minimise their difference. Morris (1991) says: 'Our bodies generally look and behave differently from most other people's (even if we have an invisible physical disability there is usually something about the way our bodies behave which gives our difference away)' (p.17).

One explanation may be that parents worked hard to give children the message that their difference had nothing to do with being of lesser value, that it was possible to be equal but different. In previous chapters, there are numerous examples of children having additional help at school, being withdrawn from their classrooms and seeing a variety of specialist staff – all of which would mark them out as different and yet, the children themselves do not name this as difference. Another part of the explanation may be that, in school, support personnel and additional equipment quickly become part of school routine (Shaw 1998) and therefore are not perceived as denoting difference. What seems to be important, then, is the management of difference.

When difference was badly managed it could lead to children experiencing hurt (pyscho-emotional damage) through being made to feel excluded or 'less than'. An older boy talked about liking the teachers in his school who treated him the same as everyone else which, by implication, means other staff behaved towards him as though he was different from the rest of his class. In Chapter 5, another older boy described how, in his school, children who used wheelchairs were made to feel different from those who were mobile. When asked how he felt about this, the boy replied: 'Sad, because we're just the same. We just can't walk, that's all the difference.'

The mother of an older boy described how he had been neglected in an emergency drill at school:

> He was telling me the other day how they did the fire alarm and every-body was screaming out in the playground. Richard was still in the school and everybody was outside. He was saying, 'Mum, I was really, really worried about what happens if there's a real fire.' No-one came to his assistance at all.

The father of a younger boy described what happened on the day of his son's school trip. His son, who had a physical impairment, wanted to travel with his peers on the bus: 'It's like he always wants to go with the class, the same on trips. He got left behind on the last trip. By the time he got to the bus, the bus was away.'

It is not known how the schools involved responded to these incidents but the latter two children were very distressed by the treatment they received – treatment which seemed almost to imply that they had less value than their peers. How do such incidents impact on children's sense of self worth? Both Morris (1991) and Thomas (1999), in their discussions with disabled adults, report the damage done to disabled people's self esteem by insensitive treatment from others. Women in Thomas's study, particularly, describe feelings of sadness, self doubt and a struggle to make sense of the negative reactions and behaviour of people around them. If such incidents are damaging to adults, it might be speculated they would be even more so to children, who are still at a relatively early stage of developing their sense of self and may be less able to rationalise their experiences.

Both the above examples suggest that when there is a change to school routine, disabled children may have to face unfortunate consequences which, at first glance, appear to be because of their difference. In reality, these consequences are the result of blanket policies, designed for the majority, which fail to take account of difference. There is also some evidence to suggest that, unless children are told why they have been placed in a particular setting – a unit or 'special' class – they may interpret their placement in a negative light. One boy described his friend thus:

Child: Because he's in a… He's like me too.

Interviewer: Like you?

Child: In the special class.

This child had become aware of his difference because he was located in a particular class in school. He then asked his parents what he had done wrong to be placed in that class. His mother replied: 'An' I said he hadnie done anything and it was just the way he was… I think when he compares himself with other children he just sees a different state and notices it.'

Why, in comparing himself with other children, did this boy feel himself to be in the wrong? How did this sense of badness or naughtiness develop? There are no clear answers from the data but perhaps, in some way, this child had learned that difference implied some kind of fault. It does suggest a need for children to have clear explanations about their schooling to minimise confusion and avoid any sense of shame.

Some children did experience their difference in positive ways. A nine-year-old boy with a physical impairment explained how he could get photographs of himself taken with various famous people because he used a wheelchair. The mother of another nine-year-old boy was told by his head teacher about his contribution to a school assembly:

I think he is quite open because he speaks up in class… There was that time, remember, when…they'd asked a question in the big hall…and he put his hand up and he went out to the front and spoke about his disability to everybody…he never told us… He never tells us anything and really we couldn't believe it. It was, 'Does anybody in here think they are special?' and he put his hand up and said, 'I am because I have cerebral palsy' and he went up to the front.

This boy was obviously secure enough in his school environment to talk about his difference, even to see his difference as something positive. At home, he rarely talked about his impairment, except when he was angry at not being able to do something but, in school, he adopted another approach altogether. It is not clear what strategies the school (a 'resourced' mainstream school) had used when working with him.

Finally, a ten-year-old deaf girl felt her hearing impairment had a number of advantages. Her mother recounted her daughter's reaction to a TV programme:

> We watched a programme the other day about Holidays from Hell…it was horrendous… They were partying till all hours…the noise was phenomenal…and Lizzie turned to me, she said, 'Well, it wouldn't bother me because I wouldn't hear them.' On another occasion she said, 'Well, if I didn't like to hear it, I'd just take my hearing aid off.'

If the management of difference, particularly the avoidance of any suggestion that it implies being of less worth, is important for the psycho-emotional well-being of disabled children, then the reactions of other people are, potentially, very damaging. The findings suggest that the young people, particularly the older group, were very aware of the unease with which they were viewed by some adults and other children. They were subjected to a variety of experiences which, even though occasional, were so distressing that they seemed to penetrate the 'immediacy' of the children's lives. The children remembered and recounted them.

REACTIONS FROM ADULTS

The older children were more likely than the younger ones to be aware of and annoyed by the attitudes and behaviour of adults. Such actions included:

- staring
- talking down, as if addressing a young child
- inappropriate comments
- inappropriate behaviour
- overt sympathy.

These could be encountered in people known to the child (in some cases, extended family members and professionals) as well as in complete strangers. A 14-year-old boy recounted a conversation he had with the school nurse who repeatedly asked if he needed to use 'nappies'. He also had to deal with a teacher who declined to talk to him but the boy chose, with great maturity, to see this as an action which was probably not deliberate: '...but I don't think he really means it. Well, I might just say it to him one day, because he's no' doing it intentionally.'

The attitudes and behaviours of strangers were just as hurtful to children. A boy who had difficulty eating disliked going out to restaurants for a meal because he was stared at:

Interviewer: Going out for a meal to restaurants and things – how do you feel about that?

Child: Stuff them. Sorry. Sorry.

Interviewer: It's okay. Don't worry about me.

Child: I don't care what they think. I used to but I try not to do it now. But you know I do. I do care. I pretend not to care but I do.

The same boy used a wheelchair and was subjected to a variety of approaches from adults because of it. People bent down to talk with him as if he was 'small' and they thought he was 'stupid'. Nevertheless, he recognised that the root of this behaviour was probably ignorance: 'Oh, I know they're just trying to help and they don't know. It's because they don't have any experience of being in a wheelchair.'

Children who used wheelchairs did seem to be a particular target for the public at large. Parents recounted a variety of incidents where misplaced sympathy – as one mother put it, an 'I'm happy I don't have to endure what you have' attitude – followed them from venue to venue. The mother of an older boy described how this could ruin a family outing:

> We go out as a family...say you go out happy, you want a nice day out and you come back thinking about all the stuff people have said to you, you know, and it really wastes your day.

Her son, however, while he was sometimes hurt after these encounters, was beginning to develop a strategy for dealing with unwanted attention. His mother gave an example:

> But he has quite a blasé attitude towards people like that now as well, which is really good. I think he said something really rude to somebody

once and I was absolutely appalled, but I said, 'That really wasn't a nice thing to say', but inside I thought 'YES'.

A number of parents described how their children seemed to be considered 'fair game' for comments or questions from strangers. The father of one girl with complex support needs met a woman whilst out shopping with his family:

> I mean there was one in Scottish Power once...she looked at Becca [the non-disabled sister] and said 'What a lovely cute wee girl you are', and then she looked at Sarah and said, 'Look at your face. What a temper. Put a smile on it.' And I said, 'She can't smile. She's got severe cerebral palsy.' She scuttled away. Nightmare, eh?

Children with less visible impairments could also attract comments from adults, usually because they were deemed to be behaving in ways which were not age appropriate. There were also issues around children getting 'special' treatment when they appeared not to need it. The father of a nine-year-old boy who had a learning impairment was annoyed when people questioned his impairment:

> I think that's one of the main problems we've got...he's classed as special needs and people have difficulty. They say, 'Why is he special needs?'... We had it when he was getting transport to school. 'Why is he getting a taxi picking him up at the door and my kid stays three, five doors away and they've got to walk (to school)?'

The mother of a ten-year-old boy also expressed frustration at the reactions of other people towards her son's 'hidden' impairment. It was her belief that a government campaign was needed to raise awareness about the issues involved.

While some children attracted too much attention from adults – they were fussed over and sometimes given money by strangers in the street – others were ignored. A boy who used sign language was not welcomed in his neighbour's house, even though other local children were. His mother felt she knew the reasons why:

> ...we had a woman who lived round the corner...and she was very anti Donald... She had said to my other neighbour, Nora, she said, 'Oh no, we're not having him in the house.' I don't know what she thought he

would do, but I think she was just so frightened of not being able to communicate with him that she didn't want him in.

REACTIONS FROM CHILDREN

There were fewer examples of children behaving in oppressive ways towards disabled children, perhaps because the two groups were less likely to have contact with each other. Many of the disabled children in the study were at schools away from their localities and thus spent little, if any, time playing with local children. However, this may also have been a cause of the name calling which seemed to be the most regular reaction of local children. As already reported, all the children subjected to this were attending schools out of their local communities. The names they were most often called were 'spassi', 'retard', 'mongol' and 'freak'.

Name calling was very upsetting for the children and liable to be deeply unsettling for them, as the mother of an older boy with a learning impairment explained:

> He was sitting day dreaming and I says, 'Are you okay, Nicky?' and he turned to me and he said, 'Am I a mongol mum?'... And I says, 'No darling, you're not.' I says, 'People might use bad words like that to describe whatever, but' I says, 'No, you're not, darling. You're Nicky, that's who you are.'

An older girl had been subjected to name calling from children at her previous place of residence. This was one of the reasons the family asked to be re-housed. These young people's experiences reflect the finding of a national study by Enable (1999) that bullying and harassment of people with learning impairments is commonplace.

Two of the younger boys had different experiences with children. One, who lived in a rural area, was blamed by local children for any misdemeanour which happened in the village. Even when he stopped playing outside, he continued to be blamed for a number of things which happened. The father of the other boy described how he had been protected by an older boy in the neighbourhood when a younger child, who was playing with water, kept trying to soak him:

> I was just watching from the window and they were soaking him...this wee boy was giving him a right soaking and the older boy came past and

grabbed hold of him and took his water pistol off and unscrewed it and emptied it across his head and said 'I don't want to catch you doing that again'.

A few children seemed unconcerned about the opinions and reactions of either adults or children. One of the younger boys was perceived, by his mother, as not one to hold a grudge. She also believed he would not know when someone was teasing him. The mother of a ten-year-old boy described how a group of local children laughed at her son when he was carrying a doll around. He did not understand their reaction:

> He thought they were trying to interact. He did not realise they were being cruel. I was hurt…but I think that's when I realised the, you know, that that's maybe one of Billy's strengths.

Both of these children had more severe learning impairments.

Most negative reactions from adults and children to disabled children were verbal. However, two girls had been abused sexually. One reported being abused by a man when she was in hospital; only her mother believed her and it took a number of years for counselling to be arranged. Eventually, this was done via a voluntary organisation of whom the girl and her mother spoke highly. The other incident was reported by a mother who believed that her daughter had been sexually abused by a boy in her mainstream school. The girl later moved to a special school which, her mother felt, suited her needs better.

Barriers to 'doing'

Various restrictions which disabled children encountered have already been discussed in Chapters 3, 4 and 5. These included the lack of access to leisure facilities and clubs, parental attitudes to children's independence, a paucity of after-school activities and, where these did take place, difficulties with transport. While a number of parents described their children as prepared 'to have a go' at most things, there were some restrictions which were hard to get beyond. These were mainly confined to physical barriers and were encountered by children who had physical impairments. Also, there was more evidence of older children being adversely affected than the younger group. The literature (Cavet 1998; Cheston 1994; Thomson *et al.* 1995) suggests that as disabled children age they encounter more physical restrictions: attempting to be more independent, they move out into the wider community and therefore experience further barriers. Also, as they grow older, parents are less able to lift and carry them.

Restrictions arose during a range of everyday activities such as getting around, shopping and eating out. Disabled children were often not able to access public transport and so either had to rely on parents to ferry them to activities or were just unable to go. Even if children managed to get to places, obstacles were often encountered therein. Lack of facilities for children suggests a number of assumptions about impairment: it is something which only 'happens' to adults, that is, it is the result of ageing, accidents or illness in later life. Alternatively, perhaps there is a belief that disabled children do not, for example, go shopping like the rest of the population. In either scenario, children were being excluded and given the message, yet again, that their lives were of lesser value.

Lack of physical access was also seen by some of the children as restrictive. The entrance and layout of such places as shops and fast food outlets was a cause for concern, as were more formal places to eat. One older boy described his feelings about having to be carried up the steps of a restaurant to take part in a family meal:

Child: ...embarrassed getting lifted up steps and that in front of everybody.

Interviewer: How does that make you feel?

Child: Angry.

Interviewer: Angry in what way?

Child: I just hate it that's all.

Interviewer: What do you do when you feel angry?

Child: Shout and swear.

Interviewer: Who do you swear at?

Child: My dad. Not in the restaurant, afterwards...he says nobody minds but they do mind...

This boy expressed his increasing dislike of going out to any restaurants – something which could, in reality, have restricted the activities of his whole family too. As already discussed, one couple was determined their ten-year-old daughter should always be included in any activity so, if places were inaccessible to her, they became inaccessible to her two non-disabled siblings as well. Another family was unable to go swimming because their nine-year-old son needed help from both parents to change. Unfortunately, the local swimming baths had no facilities for uni-sex changing. Thus, restrictions could have repercussions for whole families. A number of parents and children talked about wanting to move to the US where, they believed, there were far fewer barriers for disabled people. The mother and father of a nine-year-old boy with a physical impairment compared shopping in the US with shopping in Scotland:

Mother: ...I have seen us going to Stirling and if it is Christmas or a sale day, the shops are really inconsiderate the way they place things...there's a lot of shops I have to take him to...you cannot get him up and down the aisles because there is so much stuff.

Father: When you go in big shops in America, Jason always goes in the door and he disappears himself.

Siblings' understandings of disability

Siblings were not asked directly how they understood disability, or their brother or sister's impairment. Nevertheless, many did offer an account. This was often in response to being asked if anyone had ever spoken to them about the fact that their brother or sister could not, for example, hear or walk. Siblings tended to make the point, perhaps reflecting what they had been told, that the impairment was not the child's 'fault' but was 'the way she was born'. A few said it could not be changed; a nine-year-old girl whose brother had cerebral palsy commented that it would not get any worse but she did not know if it would get any better. A few children commented on the perceived cause of the impairment; insufficient oxygen at birth, a malfunctioning eardrum and, in one case, professional negligence:

> When she was having a baby, my mum, the nurses weren't looking what they were doing and she made her disabled. She had brain damage... (The nurses) were all too busy talking. Mum couldn't speak to them cause she had that breathing thing on her. It wasn't even fair for Poppy (the disabled child)...if she was my baby called Poppy and they made her disabled, I would (say), 'Don't you make her disabled. I just won't let you do that.'

This seven-year-old's account shows a range of feelings: a sense of injustice on her sister's behalf ('it wasn't even fair...'); absolving her mother from blame (she couldn't speak to the nurses) while at the same time implying that more could have been done to prevent the birth damage ('[the nurses] were all too busy talking...'). The confusion may have been exacerbated by the fact that the speaker was Poppy's twin, and she had not been damaged at birth.

One teenager reported that her grandparents had said the disabled child had been given to their family for a special reason, and that the family was able to look after him because they were special. The seven-year-old quoted above believed that when her twin died, she would go to heaven without any impairment:

> When all the people die are in heaven, then God makes her like us, like she can walk, she can talk, she can play in the sky. And that means we can all see the fairies, and the fairies and Jesus can look after us. But all of us who were made are the same way and Poppy isn't disabled any more, neither are we. She is just the way we are. 'Cause God made her like us.

It was not clear to what extent this girl was repeating something she had been told, confusing different things she had been told or making up her own resolution of the situation.

Other children focused on the effects of impairment. They explained that as a result of the child's condition she or he had little strength, 'gets hyper', had limited understanding, became easily frustrated, or was a slow learner. Most did not use medical terminology, although two referred to 'learning difficulties' and one to 'hypertonia'. The sibling pair who had a very poor relationship with their brother were noticeably less well informed about his impairment. They saw him as 'different' but did not know what was different about him, nor why.

Most siblings, then, focused on impairment and tended to adopt a quasi-medical model, taking an individualistic perspective and talking about the medical cause of impairment and its effects. However, it should be stressed that they did not take a 'personal tragedy' view of disability. As discussed in Chapter 6, most described their disabled brother or sister in both 'ordinary' and, overall, positive terms. It is worth adding that none of these young people saw their own position, as siblings of a disabled child, as 'tragic'.

A few older children, however, were equally aware of the social barriers associated with disability, particularly other people's negative attitudes. One teenager commented:

> I always try and work against discrimination and I wrote essays in school I felt so strongly about it, especially in like how it is in a disabled society. I don't think I would feel so strongly if I didn't have Scott.

This teenager also commented on the negative images of disabled people projected through television and other cultural media. She was one of several young people who had a strong sense of social justice and generalised from their experiences of living with a disabled sibling to the wider social context. They were well aware that the discrimination faced by their sibling also confronted many other disabled people.

Asked if having a disabled sister was different from having a non-disabled sibling, one boy replied that it was, but went on to explain this in terms of physical access. Inaccessible rides at the funfair, and difficulty pushing a wheelchair up 'hilly places' or along sandy beaches had all meant that he and his brother had been unable to pursue certain activities they wanted to. He did not attribute such restrictions to the fact that they had a disabled sister who needed parental attention (nor to his parents' management of the situation). Rather, barriers associated with physical access and the built environment were identified as the major problem.

Summary

Disabled children and their siblings had similar understandings of disability. They experienced it in terms of impairment, difference, people's reactions and physical barriers. Although impairment was usually seen in terms of a medical condition, neither group had a 'tragic' view of impairment. For the most part, they accepted it, the disabled children generally adopting a pragmatic attitude both to impairment and impairment effects. Thus, the children themselves could be said to manage difference in a practical and positive manner, usually seeing themselves as much the same as other children. They were actively choosing to make sense of their situations in a certain way. The disabled children and, to a lesser extent, their siblings could be made to feel different, however, and of lesser value, through the words and actions of others, the way difference was managed being crucial to their psycho-emotional well-being. Older disabled children were able to recount examples of people's negative reactions to them. The young people also identified restrictions on doing as they went about their everyday lives. A few disabled teenagers and older siblings talked, broadly, in terms of wider social barriers. Not surprisingly, they seemed to be more restricted than younger ones.

Chapter Eight

Conclusions

Introduction

In this chapter, we return to the original aims of the study. The first section addresses the first four aims, relating directly to disabled children and their siblings. The second part focuses on the fifth aim: to identify and draw out policy and practice implications for local authority and health services, particularly in terms of minimising the effects on children of disability and enabling them to lead as 'ordinary' lives as possible. As discussed in Chapter 1, this is directly related to the Children Act (1989), the Children (Scotland) Act 1995 and the Northern Ireland Children's Order (1995). The final section of this chapter discusses the relevance of a social model of disability for children.

Disabled children's understandings of disability

First, the study aimed to explore disabled children's understandings of disability. The findings show that they understood it through a number of concrete experiences. These experiences were mostly to do with being made to feel different through physical restrictions, institutional barriers and the reactions of others. The children never directly referred to these experiences as 'disability' (the results of an unequal social relationship); rather they were people, events and situations which, periodically, disturbed the 'ordinariness' of their everyday lives. The children also tried to make sense of the experience of impairment.

The children did not use the term 'impairment' either. They referred to it either as 'disability', 'a disability' or else in terms of a functional limitation which resulted from impairment: not being able to walk, not being able to see. Children predominantly saw impairment from a medical viewpoint or as having health implications which they had to manage. Some parents reported that they had explained impairment in terms of causation and adopted a religious angle to encourage the child to see it as part of God's 'plan'. However, the children showed agency in the management of their impairment. It was something over which they had control in their daily lives, a fact which may have encouraged their pragmatic, 'get on with it' attitude. Most seemed quite happy with themselves and their impairment, although two of them wanted to be able to walk and another wanted better vision.

In the literature, there is a strong link between the 'medical' model of disability and the notion of personal tragedy. Shakespeare and Watson (1998) talk about disabled people being portrayed as 'victims of the biomedical tragedy that is their body.' It is interesting in this study that, despite impairment being viewed, understood and often acted upon in very medical ways, no sense of tragedy was attached to it by the children, or indeed by their siblings or parents.

Parents reported that discussion with disabled children about their impairment usually arose from questions asked by the young people themselves and, once discussed, it was rarely raised again. The children themselves (unlike their brothers and sisters) did not raise this with us as a problem. It may be that some disabled children, aware or worried that further discussion could upset their parents, chose not to raise the issue of their impairment again. However, Thomas (1998), who interviewed a number of disabled women about their familial experiences, stresses the importance of on-going discussion in families about impairment. It was her conclusion that if, in the quest for 'normality', a child's experiences of impairment and disability were not acknowledged or discussed, then the consequences could be damaging.

Disabled children who attended segregated schools were more likely to talk about their impairments than those who were in other educational settings. It may be that they were used to having impairment acknowledged by those in authority, rather than avoided. One mainstream school, invited to take part in the study, declined on the grounds that use of the term 'disability' went against their policy of inclusion. Although there was no clear evidence, the children may also have been used to discussing it amongst themselves. Two children from the same school, however, either defined themselves or were defined by members of staff in terms of their impairment, suggesting practices in the school which, at the very least, were unlikely to foster a rounded self-image in the children.

Parents believed that disabled children had an awareness of themselves as different from their peers but the children themselves did not mention it. How free the children felt to describe themselves as different is not clear but if they lived in homes where discussions about impairment were restricted, and attended schools whose policies on inclusion precluded any acknowledgement of difference, then their avoidance of the topic would be understandable. For those children who attended mainstream schools, there may also have been the additional pressure of having to be the same as their peers. Indeed, Watson *et al.* (2000) argue that some disabled children who were well integrated with their peer group managed this by minimising their impairment or by passing as 'normal', neither of which was an option for most children in this study.

The ways children negotiate disability in their everyday lives

Second, the research aimed to examine how children negotiated the experience of disability in their everyday lives. The findings indicate that they did so in a very practical, matter of fact, manner. The majority declared themselves happy for most of the time; many had a sense of achievement relating to school or sports activities; all were involved in making some choices about their lives and most felt they had enough say in what was happening to them. All of this portrays disabled children as active beings who had opportunities to mould at least some aspects of their lives.

When children talked about being 'sad', this was linked to specific incidents in their lives rather than the on-going fact of impairment or the experience of disability. Many of their everyday activities and preoccupations were the same as those of non-disabled children. Any problems which they discussed tended to be in the here and now. However, boredom is a recurring theme which may be a less typical experience for children generally. Children attending schools outside their local area often reported boredom at home; many of these young people did not have friends living nearby with whom they could play. Another negative experience for some children was bullying. Almost half reported being bullied at some time in their lives either in school or in their local communities. This could be very upsetting although, in a number of cases, there were signs of agency on the part of the children – they reported the bullying behaviour to someone in authority or they took action themselves. These strategies seemed successful and the bullying did not recur. It would be wrong, however, to underestimate the effect that bullying, especially of a persistent nature, could have on some children.

Help and support from parents was very important and there was evidence of close, loving relationships. However, some parents could become over-protective in children's eyes and thus unnecessarily restrictive. This finding reflects that of Thomas (1998) who noted that as well as being 'buffers' against disablism, parents could sometimes be part of the problem. Murray (2000) also points out that over the years, parents have been 'considered to be part of the system of oppression' which affects how disabled children experience their lives (p.684), as Aspis (2000) and Campbell and Oliver (1996), for example, have argued. At the same time, Murray goes on, parents have 'described the experience of family oppression on the basis of having a disabled child', citing Murray and Penman (1996) and Rose (1997) as examples. In this study, some parents were very keen to foster independence although there were issues around how this could be managed whilst, at the same time, they were having to provide a high level of physical care for their children. A number of older children experienced this conflict as particularly frustrating.

There was also evidence of parents having a significant role in children's friendships. A more restrictive attitude on the part of parents seemed to result in children losing opportunities for friendship. Another external factor influencing friendship for children was the type of school they attended; those who travelled to schools outside their locality expressed annoyance and frustration at being able to see so little of their friends. Spending time with friends was one of the activities which made children feel happy so anything which interfered with that was bound to be viewed negatively, as were education professionals who either removed children from the company of their peers or restricted their contact. Also, there was a sense of some children being unable to control this part of their lives: they had to attend a particular school which resulted in their social lives being restricted. One boy had chosen to go to a local school to remain with his friends but, once there, experienced so much exclusion that he forfeited the opportunity to be with his friends in order to attend a segregated school in which he did not feel excluded.

School was a very important part of the children's lives. Irrespective of the type of school they attended, most were positive about it and positive about their roles there. Many described themselves as active and in control within school settings. Here, the children saw themselves as good friends, helpful classmates and active players.

Disabled children did face a number of barriers in their day to day lives. Physical restrictions were one of the main ways in which they experienced disability. These restrictions were usually around lack of accessible transport to events, inaccessible leisure facilities and diminishing social and recreational activities for older children. While there were a number of organised leisure events for the younger ones, there was nothing available to enable disabled teenagers to move from the more 'organised' leisure of their childhood to the 'casual' leisure of adolescence (Cavet 1998). The latter has been described as boys hanging around in groups outside and girls congregating in bedrooms (Cavet 1998), neither of which might be possible for some disabled adolescents. Since adolescence has been described as the peak time of leisure need (Hendry et al. 1993) then the exclusion of disabled teenagers could have serious consequences for their social well-being.

Looking towards the future, most of the older children believed they would be employed and were content to work for qualifications at school to ensure this. However, one boy doubted he would get a job because the prevailing work culture was not accepting of disabled people. In turn, this influenced his thinking about working for exams at school and getting a place in college. Other young people talked about not being able to do certain jobs because their impairment mitigated against working in a number of professions. It was not clear where the children's information about disabled people at work had come from. There did not seem to be any evidence of contact with disabled adults who were in employment and who would be able to provide role models for young disabled people as they made decisions about their future.

Children's experiences of services and professionals

A third aim of the research was to examine the children's perceptions of their relationships with professionals, and their knowledge and views of service provision. While they did not identify as wide a range of professionals with whom they had contact as their parents did, they were, on the whole, positive in their views. As a group, they had a high level of contact with medical professionals and significant experience of hospital admissions. These were not seen as pleasant experiences. Sometimes, children's wards were not geared up for disabled children, for example, lacking accessible toilets, and there were incidences of children having to argue with professionals before they were listened to. There were also examples of children being dealt with in creative and sensitive ways. Generally, however, health professionals seemed to be distant figures for the children. There was some confusion in their minds about consultants and GPs and little willingness to comment in depth upon them. It may be that, since most doctors were not seen on a daily basis and therefore not part of the 'immediacy' of the children's lives, little attention was paid to them. More attention was paid, by some of the children, to physiotherapists. They tended to be seen regularly and their treatments were, in some cases, the cause of discomfort for the children. Occupational therapists, whilst seen less regularly and by few children, were perceived as helpful because they could obtain equipment.

Children seemed to be most positive about education professionals, perhaps because they had a great deal of contact with them. They spoke well of their class teacher if they were in primary schools, or at least one of their teachers if in secondary schools. The majority of conflict with school staff seemed to focus on special needs assistants who sometimes acted as a barrier between children and their peers. This is undoubtedly a key role in schools and the policy implications will be discussed later in the chapter.

Short breaks for disabled children was a more problematic area. One child had a particularly positive experience at her 'hotel' with carefully planned, regular visits. For a number of others, there was no such planning and whilst they reported that they enjoyed the experience, it was not regular enough. The two children with complex needs went into a local children's ward for regular short breaks. Their parents felt that they did not enjoy the experience and, using non-verbal communication, made their displeasure known. One child commented on her social worker. She said that she rarely saw her. The other children who had contact with social workers seemed not to know who they were.

The children's involvement with voluntary organisations seemed to be more positive. Not only was there more frequent contact between them, but also they provided opportunities for leisure, some peer support and, when needed, specialist services such as counselling.

Siblings' views and experiences

A fourth aim of the study was to explore siblings' views of the effects on them of having a disabled brother or sister. Most seemed to perceive the relationship in predominantly positive terms, although there were a small number of exceptions. There was a large reciprocal element in many of the relationships and, interestingly, some of the siblings' descriptions confound a number of stereotypes about the implications of specific impairments. Siblings described relationships in which there was some conflict, much of which seemed to be 'normal' bickering between brothers and sisters. Some also seemed happy to acknowledge and accept their disabled sibling as different. Others did not see anything different about their brother or sister. When difference was noted, however, it was seldom reported as being 'lesser'. It was not something to be worked on, to be removed or to be 'normalised'; rather, it was viewed as being an integral part of the child, which was in keeping with disabled children's own views of themselves. The exceptions were the few cases of problematic relationships, where it seems the disabled child was primarily seen as 'bad'.

Siblings talked about the causes of impairment in either physiological or religious terms. It had happened through, perhaps, a combination of factors including illness or complications at birth, or as part of a plan that 'God' had for the family. Thus, the presence of impairment was not something over which families had any control. At the same time, many children wanted to find out more about the implications of their sister or brother's impairment: to ask questions, discuss worries and seek reassurance. Without this, as Tozer (1996) points out, some siblings may invent their own diagnoses and prognoses. In a number of cases, parents thought they had informed siblings sufficiently about the disabled child's impairment and believed that discussion in the family was quite open, but their children were actually wanting more opportunity to ask questions or talk. Some siblings perceived their parents as discouraging or fearful of further discussion.

Alongside the positive feelings siblings reported for their disabled sister or brother there were some frustrations and resentments. These seemed to focus on two areas: other people's attitudes and parental preoccupation with the disabled child. In fact, only a small number of children identified effects in any particular area of their lives, a finding which differs from some of the literature (Baldwin and Carlisle 1994; Wheeler 1993). The difference can be explained in two ways: first, siblings were asked to give their own accounts and, second, the wording of the questions did not assume a negative response. It is noticeable that parental accounts were more qualified.

A number of siblings described being bullied because of their disabled sister or brother and talked of ways in which they tried to manage it. However, several had not told anyone in authority and were attempting to cope with the situation without support. Some of them had done so over a number of years. It may be that not telling parents about bullying was a further attempt to protect or avoid upsetting them. Alternatively, a 'don't talk' rule may have been operating in some families whereby children felt unable to discuss any aspect of disability, including the fact that the presence of their disabled brother or sister resulted in them being bullied in school. Mellor (1990) noted the great 'taboo' against reporting bullying in mainstream Scottish schools. In his study, the children who did report bullying were more likely to tell their parents than teachers, which suggests there may be a doubly difficult situation for bullied siblings of disabled children. Those who would feel more comfortable telling parents about bullying could be constrained from doing so through fear of upsetting them or to avoid breaking the 'don't talk' rule. There was also evidence of teachers not being aware that children in their care had a disabled sibling. If parents chose not to share such information with school staff, then it follows that their non-disabled children could feel compelled to keep the secret too and so, should bullying occur in school, feel themselves forced to keep silent about it.

Nearly all the siblings interviewed said that they worried about their disabled brother or sister. Much of their concern centred on health and physical well-being, including worries about the long-term prognosis for children who had more serious conditions. Another area of concern was to do with disabled children being bullied or taken advantage of, which is interesting given that disabled children were more likely to report bullying than their siblings. However, much of this concern stemmed from a perception of the disabled child as being potentially vulnerable, although some siblings had witnessed their brother or sister being ill-treated.

Policy and practice implications

That disabled children and their siblings in this study already managed to lead fairly 'ordinary' lives is as much a testament to their tenacity and that of their parents as it is to the quality of support offered them. The data suggest a number of areas where that support might be improved.

Communication

Some families undoubtedly encouraged clear communication about impairment but many did not. Promoting a culture of openness in families about impairment is a very challenging goal and would need to be tackled, it seems, in different ways as children grow up. Many parents described how some professionals had behaved in deeply insensitive ways at the time of their child's diagnosis, adding to the distress of the occasion and, perhaps, helping to create a reluctance to talk about the child. These data have not been presented in previous chapters because they did not relate directly to the child's experience, and similar experiences around the time of birth and diagnosis have been well documented elsewhere (Jupp 1992; Mason 1995; Murray 2000). It is well established that the right support is crucial at this time and this calls for a partnership between health professionals, social services and voluntary agencies. The latter often have particular expertise in peer support. The importance of providing good support to parents at the point of diagnosis is reiterated here because it could be of great benefit in encouraging parents to have the confidence to communicate about impairment more openly with their children as they grow up.

Tozer (1996) suggests that at diagnosis, thought should also be given to the needs of siblings and how to explain the child's impairment to them. Again, voluntary agencies could be utilised to provide either groups for children or one to one counselling. Some siblings involved in the study were clear about the importance of talking to someone their own age who had similar experiences; thus there is a role for peer support also. Clearly, there is a need for a range of options to be available so that individual children can choose what, if anything (not all siblings wanted support), suits them best. It may be that siblings will need different types of support as they get older. There is also a need for support to siblings and parents to be resourced properly; Tozer (1996) notes that many voluntary groups run on a shoestring.

Disabled children seemed not to be talking to anyone about their impairments or any of the barriers they faced. Young disabled people in the study by Beresford and Sloper (2000) reported that one of the most useful sources of information and support was other young people of similar ages with the same condition whom they wanted to meet in informal social settings. However, they had few opportunities for contact with peers in similar circumstances. Children in this study also had few opportunities to meet disabled peers in social settings; those who attended segregated and integrated schools often had great difficulty socialising because of transport problems. Children in inclusive settings were often the only disabled child in their school, a number of which seemed to have policies designed to minimise or even deny the fact that they had impairments at all. So how could disabled children get in touch with their peers? Beresford and Sloper (2000) suggest a number of ways to establish contact between young disabled people. As well as group and one to one meetings, there could also be telephone, email or Internet contact – some or all of which could be facilitated by schools and voluntary organisations, with adequate resources, working together.

Bullying

The bullying of some disabled children and their siblings in schools and local neighbourhoods is a cause for concern. Whilst it is positive that most of the children took action to stop the bullying from recurring, questions still need to be asked about the effectiveness of anti-bullying strategies in schools. Schools could do more to encourage parents to tell teachers where there is a disabled child in the family; similarly, staff need to be made aware that this can sometimes be a trigger for siblings to be bullied, and to look out for signs that it may be happening.

The bullying of both siblings and disabled children is also linked to a wider issue about public attitudes and thus the need for better public education. Recommendation 21 of the Scottish Executive Review (2000) of services to people with learning disabilities recommended a long-term programme to promote public awareness about people with learning disabilities and strategies for including them in the community. Part of this programme, the Review said, should be implemented from the earliest years of education. The Scottish Consortium for Learning Disability is charged with taking forward this task. There is no equivalent initiative in England.

Services

SHORT BREAKS

The picture which emerges of short breaks is depressing, not least because much previous research has produced similar results (see, for example, reviews by Robinson 1996, and Russell 1996b). Children and their parents were clear about what they wanted. Disabled children wanted to have more frequent short breaks (although some of that was linked to having little to occupy them at home) where they could do interesting things. Parents also wanted regular breaks, which offered good quality care and an opportunity for their child to do something creative, something which would add to their lives. Siblings wanted to have time with their parents while feeling confident that their disabled sister or brother was happy. Therefore, it is crucial to provide short breaks which suit the whole family.

Robinson (1996) highlighted innovative forms of short breaks from the UK, Scandinavia, Australia and the US. They included:

- Befriending services: schemes which offer an opportunity for young people to go out with a friend on a regular basis and become involved in activities which interest them both.

- Outreach services: these began as residential services but gradually moved towards providing a range of weekend and evening activities where staff support young people when they attend local groups such as Brownies, youth clubs and evening classes. This enables children to develop links with their communities. Staff also take children away on holiday or, if needed, accompany families on holiday to share caring for the young person.

- Co-operative sitting: a service where families with disabled children care for other disabled children on a reciprocal basis so that children are not moved out of their home environments. Potential families are given training before such schemes are set up.

- Summer camps: in Sweden, disabled children attend summer camps for three-week periods and while many of these are segregated, inclusive camps are becoming available. Children tend to return to the same camp every year so workers get to know them very well. Friends and other family members are offered the opportunity to accompany the child.

- After-school services: disabled children are able to participate in local childcare services before and after school and in school holidays, which not only provides support and encourages inclusion in existing services, but also enables parents to take paid employment if they so wish.

- Specialist child-minders: a scheme whereby child-minders are given specialist training to care for disabled children, so providing the chance for parents to return to work. Ideally, these child-minders also take non-disabled children.

When a number of the above strategies are available on a regular basis, the need for residential placements is reduced (Robinson 1996). Thus, the stress and anxiety which residential breaks seem to induce in families would also be reduced.

There may be other approaches which would suit some families. One of the teenaged siblings in the study suggested that more help within the home would free up his parents to spend time with their non-disabled children. However, he made the point that he would not want these people in the house all of the time because 'We'd never get any peace or anything.'

HEALTH

Families reported a number of unhelpful and hurtful experiences with GPs. In their view, good practice from a GP included the following:

- building up a relationship with the child over time
- speaking directly to the child, using appropriate language
- if the child had no speech or was reluctant to speak, the doctor still addressed her/him directly
- seeing the child as an individual, not an impairment
- every minor illness the child contracted was not seen as being linked to the child's impairment.

Some of the GPs whom families valued also had personal family experience of impairment. The young disabled people interviewed by Beresford and Sloper (2000) had very similar views of what constituted good practice among doctors. These findings have implications for the initial and on-going training of GPs.

Other health professionals – physiotherapists, occupational, speech and language therapists – were also the focus of some criticism. Children and parents felt that some physiotherapists could be more sensitive in their dealings with families. They wanted them to listen to both children and adults and be prepared to work in partnership. Occupational therapists, while seen as helpful, were not being proactive. Families seemed to initiate contact with them which suggests little long-term planning was taking place and no attempt to pre-empt difficulties. There were too few speech and language therapists working with disabled children, resulting in long gaps in the service offered when personnel moved on to other positions. For all of these professionals there are training and recruitment implications.

EDUCATION

Parents reported a higher level of contact with inclusive schools than either integrated or segregated schools. While local education authorities may have clear policies about inclusion, there is evidence to suggest that these have yet to be fully accepted by some schools. Overall, the picture which emerges is of a few schools welcoming disabled children and working hard to facilitate inclusion, a number of others where staff opposition, either covert or overt, made inclusion almost impossible, and a group in the middle which seemed happy to include but had only rudimentary knowledge about what this meant in terms of policy, personnel and training. Thus, it is crucial that the principle of inclusion is embedded within every aspect of school policy, rather than being a 'stand alone' item with little effect on either day to day operations or overall ethos.

Several of the mainstream schools approached in the early stages of this project appeared to misunderstand the philosophy of inclusion. For them it seemed to revolve around minimising difference, avoiding discussion of impairment and a desire never to single out disabled children. To adopt such an approach may, initially, satisfy a very superficial notion of inclusion but it fails to address deeper issues, notably those around educating children to accept and respect difference. The result of such a failure could be an increase in intolerance and bullying. Davis and Watson (2001) argue that although much attention is, rightly, focused on removing structural barriers to inclusion, what they call 'personal and institutional cultural values' must also be addressed. Murray (2000) argues that schools must shift from seeing disability in terms of individual deficit to 'embracing equality of value for all':

> Our experience was that it was only possible for partnerships to be formed when professionals, while simultaneously doing their very best for my son, were able to value and enjoy him without wanting him to change in order that he fit into the current education system. (p.696)

Integrated units and segregated schools have their own particular difficulties. For the most part, children in integrated settings were not being included with their peers at any point during their school day. Indeed, on some occasions, they were not even to be found in the same playground, with the result that many of the children attending units were really in segregated settings. Why are children in these units at all, if there is no attempt to include them in mainstream? Nor was it clear how such practice linked with schools' policies on inclusion. It would appear there is some questionable practice being undertaken in segregated schools. The children described it and were distressed by it. Children being further segregated according to impairment suggests the presence of, and practice related to, a medical model of disability with little, if any, understanding of a social model. In turn, this suggests a dearth of contact with disability organisations and disabled role models for the children, which may not benefit their development.

The issue of children's friendships outside integrated and segregated settings needs to be a concern of schools. Children who have to travel to school require support and opportunities to maintain social lives related to school but outside of school hours.

The data suggest there are a number of implications for training at various levels:

- Management: the role of the head teacher is pivotal for the success of inclusion. Head teachers giving a strong lead in the creation of a culture of inclusion and acceptance of difference are invaluable in any school, yet such individuals were rarely encountered by parents in the study. Thus, training about inclusion, preferably involving organisations of disabled people, should be an essential part of the route towards any management role in schools.

- School staff: teachers and special needs assistants (SNAs) have particular training needs around both inclusion and disability awareness, again involving disabled adults. For the former there are issues of classroom management as well as work organisation; for the latter, whose role requires both sensitivity and awareness, there is a need for careful selection, supervision and on-going training. The UK Local Government National Training Organisation has recently developed national occupational standards for all paid staff working with teachers in the classroom, including SNAs. Both Watson *et al.* (2000) and Shaw (1998) stress the centrality of the SNAs' role in the inclusion of disabled children. Skar and Tamm (2001) report that children appreciated assistants who see them 'as the persons they are and ignored their disabilities' (p.928). The young people were better able to develop as individuals when they felt they were on a more equal footing with their assistant, and there was mutual respect. Staff in segregated schools need the opportunity to develop understandings of social theories of disability.

- Pupils: the pupils' role in the success of inclusion is also important. Shaw (1998) describes the positive reactions of non-disabled children to the inclusion of disabled children in mainstream schools and how, as children grew up together, acceptance increased and friendships flourished. Opportunities to learn about and discuss difference, along with input from disabled adults, would help to create openness about diversity.

It is worth adding that this research was completed prior to the passing of the Standards in Scotland's Schools Etc. Act 2000. This legislation includes a presumption of mainstream schooling for all children. The Special Educational Needs & Disability Act 2001 (SENDA), which applies to England, Wales and Scotland and comes into force from 2002, extends the Disability Discrimination Act 1995 to education.

SENDA places two key duties on education providers. First, they must not treat disabled pupils, or potential pupils, less favourably than any others. Second, they must make reasonable adjustments to ensure disabled pupils do not face substantial disadvantage. In addition, the Education (Disability Strategies and Pupils' Educational Records) (Scotland) Bill requires responsible bodies to publish and implement accessibility strategies in schools. This means that local authorities will need to be proactive in their planning for disabled pupils rather than making support available as and when required by the arrival of an individual disabled child (Riddell 2002), as was sometimes the case in this study.

SOCIAL WORK

Most of the parents who had contact with social work services viewed them in a negative light. This was particularly true of the small number of parents with allocated social workers who were seen as knowing very little about disabled children. At no time was there a sense of partnership between parents and social work professionals.

This lack of partnership is unfortunate since a major gap in the lives of the families seemed to be the absence of a professional to co-ordinate services for them. There is clear evidence (Beresford *et al.* 1996; Mukherjee, Beresford and Sloper 1999) that having a key worker has a beneficial effect and yet none of the families in the study had such support. Again, the situation should improve for families whose children have learning disabilities because, following the recent national reviews of services (Scottish Executive 2000; DoH 2001), steps are being taken to improve co-ordination. In Scotland, local area co-ordinators are being appointed for every family. In England, £60 million from the *Quality Protects* programme has been earmarked, from 2001–2004, for families with disabled children, with a focus on providing more access to key workers. The extension of direct payments to families with disabled children opens up possibilities for some parents to act as their own 'key worker'. For a variety of reasons, however, this will not be an appropriate option for some families.

In the final section of this chapter, we move on to look at the study's implications for the relevance of a social model of disability to children.

Children and a social model of disability

'Children' is no more a unifying concept than 'men' or 'women'. Variables including gender, age and cultural issues bring much to bear on the everyday lives of disabled children and their siblings in ways which it has not been possible to explore in this study. However, as an early piece of work in what, it must be assumed, will be the developing field of child-hood disability studies, this research has a role in identifying themes and issues which may be explored later in more depth. Key themes to emerge from this study of children's daily lives include:

- the 'ordinariness' of children's lives
- their perceptions of impairment
- their understandings of difference
- children's friendships
- the 'ordinariness' of sibling relationships
- the agency of disabled children
- their positive outlook overall
- communication within families.

Thomas's (1999) social relational model of disability was developed primarily with adults in mind but seems to fit well with the children's accounts of their everyday lives. It is not, of course, being suggested that the children themselves understood their situation according to Thomas's framework; rather, that this framework helps to explain different aspects of their experiences and their interrelation. Most children were aware of their *impairment*, which they saw primarily in medical and functional terms, and they talked about *impairment effects* – the things they could not do because of their impairment, or the fact that they sometimes felt fatigue or discomfort as a result of having an impairment. We have already discussed why children may have focused on the medical or health implications of impairment, but it is important to stress that they did not adopt a personal tragedy view of disability, often associated with the medical model. Most accepted impairment and got on with their lives in as ordinary a way as they could.

There was much evidence of *disability* in the children's accounts; that is, *barriers to being*, such as the thoughtless or hostile attitudes and behaviour of others, as well as *barriers to doing*: of the material, structural and institutional kind. The former was probably more dominant than the latter in the children's narratives and, we have suggested, may have a particularly far-reaching effect, perhaps more so than on adults. Thus, in considering the relevance to children of a social relational model, 'barriers to being' may take on heightened significance.

We have also seen how there may be repercussions for those around the disabled child, particularly her/his brothers and sisters. In particular, siblings who were bullied or teased, and the teenager whose boyfriends deserted her, could be said to experience damage to their psycho-emotional well-being. It is not possible to draw conclusions about the nature or extent of the damage that may be done, and perhaps it would be invidious to try to 'compare' its impact to that experienced by the disabled children. On the one hand, where siblings were teased, it was only about one aspect of their lives: having a disabled brother or sister. On the other hand, the hurtful comments made could, of course, be aimed at their 'whole person'.

Some siblings also reported restrictions on their activities, such as the brothers who, because of their parents' determination to include their disabled daughter in all family activities, were not able to go to certain places or do certain things that were not fully accessible. Dowling and Dolan (2001) have argued that whole families can experience unequal opportunities and outcomes; these authors draw on the social model to illustrate how families with disabled children often face financial hardship, stress and anxiety.

Can we relate the present findings about siblings and parents to Thomas's reworking of the social model? There are dangers in isolating parts of her framework in order to argue that one element 'fits' or can be applied to siblings or parents, since the framework is a complex one, in which each part gains meaning from its interaction with the other elements. Most siblings and parents do not have impairments and thus, it could be argued, their experiences have no place in the framework nor can it be related to them. Here again the notion of difference, and the extent to which disabled people are or are not different from others, is crucial. We would argue that most children are likely to 'feel' and react to bullying and taunting in broadly similar ways – or, at the least, that the presence of impairment will not be a distinguishing factor in their responses.

The findings suggest that the impact of psycho-emotional attacks on siblings are similar to the felt experience of disabled children, although they probably affect far fewer numbers of siblings and may have a different longer term impact, although we do not know this. Where siblings and parents face restrictions of activity, the findings show that this is due to a combination of factors, some of which families may have little control over, such as their financial circumstances and lack of appropriate or available formal support. There are other aspects over which they may have more control, such as the way parents choose to manage certain situations. In fact, parents and siblings have a potentially ambiguous role, since they may also contribute to barriers to being and doing affecting the disabled child, acting, in Thomas's phrase, as 'carriers' or 'agents' of disablism.

The attitudes and responses of other people seemed to have a huge influence on disabled children's perception of their difference. The majority of reported responses were negative and could range from mis-placed sympathy to cruelty. Reactions such as those described by some of the children and the majority of their parents would be unlikely to result in children viewing difference as positive. The young people showed a variety of responses which suggested that they had mechanisms for dealing with unwanted and negative attention. In the first place, there was the recognition that people's behaviour was, generally, an outcome of ignorance. This gave children the choice of showing sympathy and under-standing towards such acts of ignorance. It also gave them a degree of control in the situation: they had choices about how to behave. Another option was to confront the unwanted attention immediately with some kind of verbal response. The children's behaviour in these instances reflected agency, not passivity.

For the professionals involved, difference seemed to be something to be removed, minimised and, in some situations, denied altogether. Health professionals worked to produce as much 'normal' functioning as possible. Most educationalists expected difference to be minimised – if it were not and disabled children began to 'fall behind' their non-disabled peers, then action was taken. This was often action to segregate children on the grounds that it was for their own good. Thus, there did not seem to be a positive approach to difference in a number of the services disabled children encountered, some of which seemed to be working out of a 'deficit' model. Nor did there seem to be any attempt among some services to educate themselves, other children, or the public in general about the value of difference.

Disabled children were made to feel different when they came up against institutional discrimination, often in schools. None of this seemed to be deliberate on the part of the schools; rather it was a result of policies being constructed on the assumption that all children were without impairments. The resulting exclusion, however, gave children, and their parents, the message that they were of less worth or value than other children.

In the light of the negativity which surrounded disabled children it is surprising that siblings viewed their disabled brothers and sisters in other ways altogether. Some were aware of their disabled sisters and brothers as different but this difference was not usually seen as detrimental. Rather, they were prepared to look at the strengths of their disabled brother or sister. Throughout many of the siblings' accounts was the sense of their sister or brother being different but, nevertheless, equal. This has much in common with the 'essentialist' view of difference espoused by some disabled academics and writers, outlined in Chapter 1.

How did siblings come to these conclusions about their disabled brothers and sisters? This is not clear from the data. Some parents did have very empowering attitudes towards their disabled children, encouraging them to be independent and to make choices about their lives. However, there was significant evidence of communication difficulties around the issue of impairment in a number of families, with siblings wanting the freedom to ask more questions but viewing their parents as unwilling or unhappy about providing answers.

For some of the older siblings there seemed to be an awareness of disability – the social restrictions encountered by their brothers and sisters. This was particularly evident, they felt, in other people's negative attitudes and the negative ways in which disabled people are portrayed in the media. A number of these teenagers seemed to have developed a strong sense of social justice and an understanding of the discrimination faced by disabled people as a whole.

The views of disabled children themselves are even more intriguing. While they were regularly treated as though they were different, the children rarely, if ever, described themselves as such. Parents believed that most of them felt themselves to be different but this (as with other issues around impairment) seemed not to have been discussed in any detail. Watson *et al.* (2000) note that social settings and adult behaviour are instrumental in the creation of disability as a separate category. The ways in which adults discussed disabled children, the way that 'social space' was organised and the ways in which other differences were minimised all served to remind children of their difference. The same processes were in operation for the children in this study, but their refusal to categorise themselves as different or as part of a distinct group – the adoption of a 'we're the same, we just happen to use wheelchairs' attitude – suggests other influences may be at work. This also chimes with the notion of difference being socially constructed.

It may, of course, be necessary for some children to deny their difference. Thomas (1998) encountered a number of women in her study for whom the pursuit of 'normality' was part of a family goal from which they deviated at their peril. Structures within schools (Shaw 1998) are designed to make even the most obvious of help/support, which would suggest difference, subsumed as part of an unrelenting routine. Watson *et al.* (2000) report children who minimise difference to be accepted and to fit in. Some inclusive schools avoid use of the term 'disability' at all. Denial of difference could be a dominant issue for many disabled children. However, what if the issue is less one of denial and more to do with not having a language with which to discuss difference?

Thomas (1999) describes the importance of 'counter-narrative' as a critique of dominant public narratives. That is, people who are excluded from mainstream society tell their own story. In so doing, they not only offer a criticism of the mainstream but also encourage others to identify with their story and, as a result, attempt to change the major narrative. In this way a new social movement becomes possible. The presence of a social model of disability offers a counter-narrative; disabled people have been able to construct narratives which have encouraged other disabled people to identify with these new narratives and, collectively, work for change. However, children's narratives are lacking in this process. Disabled children have almost no opportunities to hear the stories of disabled adults and the Disability Rights Movement as a whole, nor to tell each other about their lives. Without this framework for making sense of their lives, children have few choices other than to strive to be the same as their non-disabled peers.

For the children's narratives to be heard and engaged with, there is need for a social model of disability which is open to the role of experience. If children are to share, with each other and with disabled adults, the fabric of their lives and the ways in which the actions and reactions of others restrict not only their activities but also their sense of self, they need a community of disabled people, including academics, ready to hear them. They also need a society which is ready to accept and value difference; they need to encounter professionals who are willing to recognise the positive in difference and be part of families who are not afraid to discuss difference. The implications of this for those who work with disabled children and their families are enormous.

References

Abberley, P. (1987) 'The concept of oppression and the development of a social theory of disability.' *Disability, Handicap and Society 2*, 5–19.

Abbot, D., Morris, J. and Ward, L. (2001) *The Best Place To Be? Policy, Practice and the Experience of Residential School Placements for Disabled Children.* York: Joseph Rowntree Foundation, York Publishing Services.

Alderson, P. (1995) *Listening to Children: Children, Ethics and Social Research.* Barkingside: Barnardos.

Anderson, D. (1997) *The Family Link Scheme – A Retrospective Study.* Dundee: Barnardos Family Support Team.

Ash, A., Bellew, J., Davies, M., Newman, T. and Richardson, L. (1996) *Everybody In? The Experience of Disabled Students in Colleges of Further Education.* Barkingside: Barnardos.

Aspis, S. (2001) 'Inclusive education – disabled children's issues and rights.' In P. Murray and J. Penman (eds) *Telling Our Own Stories – Reflections on Family Life in a Disabling World.* Sheffield: Parents with Attitude.

Baldwin, S. and Carlisle, J. (1994) *Social Support for Disabled Children and their Families: A Review of the Literature.* Edinburgh: HMSO.

Beresford, B. (1994) *Positively Parents: Caring for a Severely Disabled Child.* London: HMSO/SPRU.

Beresford, B. (1997) *Personal Accounts: Involving Disabled Children in Research.* London: HMSO/SPRU.

Beresford, B. and Sloper, P. (2000) *The Information Needs of Chronically Ill or Physically Disabled Children and Adolescents.* York: Social Policy Research Unit, University of York.

Beresford, B., Sloper, P., Baldwin, S. and Newman, T. (1996) *What Works in Services for Families with a Disabled Child?* Barkingside: Barnardos.

Bersoff, D. and Hofer, P. (1990) 'The legal regulation of school psychology.' In J. Gutkin and C. Reynolds (eds) *The Handbook of Social Psychology.* New York: Wiley.

Bignall, T. and Butt, J. (2000) *Between Ambition and Achievement: Young Black Disabled People's Views of Independence and Independent Living.* York: Joseph Rowntree Foundation.

Brannen, J. and O'Brien, M. (1995) 'Childhood and the sociological gaze: Paradigms and paradoxes.' *Sociology 29*, 4, 729–737.

Brazier, M. and Lobjoit, M. (1991) *Protecting the Vulnerable: Autonomy and Consent in Health Care.* London: Routledge.

Campbell, J. and Oliver, M. (1996) *Disability Politics: Understanding our Pasts, Changing our Futures.* London: Routledge.

Carers' (Recognition and Services) Act (1995). London: HMSO.

Cavet, J. (1995) *Interviewing Children and Young People with Chronic Health Conditions: Some Issues for Researchers.* (Unpublished paper), School of Social Science, Staffordshire University.

Cavet, J. (1998) 'Leisure and friendship.' In C. Robinson and K. Stalker (eds) *Growing Up with Disability.* Research Highlights in Social Work Series, London: Jessica Kingsley Publishers.

Cheston, R. (1994) 'The accounts of special education leavers.' *Disability and Society 9,* 1, 59–69.

Children Act (1989). London: HMSO.

Children (Northern Ireland) Order (1995). Belfast: The Stationery Office.

Children (Scotland) Act (1995). Edinburgh: HMSO.

Children and Society 11 (1997) Special edition on 'Communicating with Children.'

Children in Scotland (2000) *Consulting with Children whose Impairments Affect their Communication.* Special Needs Forum, Factsheet 1, Edinburgh: Children in Scotland.

Closs, A. (1998) 'Quality of life for children and young people with serious medical conditions.' In C. Robinson and K. Stalker (eds) *Growing Up with Disability.* Research Highlights in Social Work Series, London: Jessica Kingsley Publishers.

Cocks, E. and Cockran, J. (1995) 'The participatory research paradigm and intellectual disability.' *Mental Handicap Research 8,* 25–37.

Crow, L. (1996) 'Including all of our lives: Renewing the social model of disability.' In C. Barnes and G. Mercer (eds) *Exploring the Divide: Illness and Disability.* Leeds: The Disability Press.

Davis, J. M. and Watson N. (2001) 'Where are the children's experiences? Analysing social and cultural exclusion in "special" and "mainstream" school.' *Disability and Society 16,* 5, 671–687.

Department of Health (1998)*Quality Protects: Framework for Action.* London: The Stationery Office.

Department of Health (2001) *Valuing People: A New Strategy for Learning Disability for the 21st Century.* A White Paper, Cm 5086, London: HMSO.

Disability Discrimination Act (1995). Norwich: HMSO.

Dowling, M. and Dolan, L. (2001) 'Disabilities – inequalities and the social model.' *Disability and Society 16,* 1, 21–36.

Education (Disability Strategy and Pupil's Educational Records) (Scotland) Act (2002). Norwich: HMSO.

Enable/Mencap/VIA (1999) *STOP IT! Bullying and Harassment of People with Learning Disabilities.* Glasgow: Enable.

Finkelstein, V. (1980) *Attitudes and Disabled People: Issues for Discussion.* New York: World Rehabilitation Fund.

Finkelstein, V. (1996) 'Outside, inside out.' *Coalition,* April, 30–36.

Finkelstein, V. and French, S. (1993) 'Towards a psychology of disability.' In J. Swain, V. Finkelstein, S. French and M. Oliver (eds) *Disabling Barriers – Enabling Environments.* London: Sage.

Flynn, M. and Hirst, M. (1992) *This Year, Next Year, Sometime? Learning Disability and Adulthood.* London/York: National Development Team/SPRU.

Glendinning, C. (1983) *Unshared Care: Parents and their Disabled Children.* London: Routledge and Kegan Paul.

Hames, A. (1998) 'Do the younger siblings of learning-disabled children see them as similar or different?' In *Child: Care, Health and Development 24,* 2, 157–168.

Hazel, N. (1996) 'Elicitation techniques with young people.' *Sociology at Surrey 12,* Spring, University of Surrey.

Hendry, L. B., Shucksmith, J., Love, J. G. and Glendinning, A. (1993) *Young People's Leisure and Lifestyles.* London: Routledge.

Hevey, D. (1993) 'The tragedy principle: strategies for change in the representation of disabled people.' In J. Swain, V. Finkelstein, S. French and M. Oliver (eds) *Disabling Barriers – Enabling Environments.* London: Sage.

Hirst, M. and Baldwin, S. (1994) *Unequal Opportunities: Growing Up Disabled.* London: HMSO.

James, A. (1993) *Childhood Identities: Self and Social Relationships in the Experience of the Child.* Edinburgh: Edinburgh University Press.

James, A. and Prout, A. (eds) (1997) *Constructing and Reconstructing Childhood: Contemporary Issues in the Sociological Study of Childhood.* London: Falmer.

Jupp, S. (1992) *Making the Right Start.* Hyde: Opened Eye.

Kelly, B., McColgan, M. and Scally, M. (2000) 'A chance to say: Involving children who have learning disabilities in a pilot study on family support services.' *Journal of Learning Disabilities 4,* 2, 115–127.

Kosonen, M. (1996) 'Siblings as providers of support and care during middle childhood: children's perceptions.' *Children and Society 10,* 267–279.

Laybourn, A. and Cutting, E. (1996) *Young People with Epilepsy: Supports and Services Existing and Desired: Research Study for Enlighten, Final Report.* University of Glasgow, Centre for the Child and Society.

Lobato, D. J. (1990) *Brothers and Sisters with Special Needs: Information and Activities for Helping Young Siblings of Children with Chronic Illnesses and Developmental Disabilities.* Baltimore: Paul H. Brookes.

McCormack, M. (1978) *A Mentally Handicapped Child in the Family.* London: Constable.

Macaskill, C. (1985) *Against the Odds: Adopting Mentally Handicapped Children.* London: British Agencies for Adoption and Fostering.

Macklin, R. (1992) 'Autonomy, beneficence and child development: An ethical analysis.' In B. Stanley and J. E. Sieber (eds) *Social Research on Children and Adolescents: Ethical Issues.* California: Sage.

Mason, M. (1995) 'Breaking of relationships.' *Present Time,* January, 3–7.

Mellor, A. (1990) 'Bullying in Scottish secondary schools.' *Spotlights,* The Scottish Council for Research in Education.

Meltzer, H., Smyth, M. and Robins, N. (1989) 'Disabled children: Services, transport and education.' *OPCS Surveys of Disability in Great Britain Report 6.* London: HMSO.

Minkes, J., Robinson, C. and Weston, C. (1994) 'Consulting the children: interviews with children using residential respite care services.' *Disability and Society 9,* 1, 47–56.

Morris, J. (1991) *Pride against Prejudice: Transforming Attitudes to Disability.* London: The Women's Press.

Morris, J. (1993) 'Gender and disability.' In J. Swain, V. Finkelstein, S. French and M. Oliver (eds) *Disabling Barriers – Enabling Environments.* London: Sage.

Morris, J. (1995) *Gone Missing? A Research and Policy Review of Disabled Children Living Away from their Families.* London: Who Cares? Trust.

Morris, J. (ed) (1996) *Encounters with Strangers: Feminism and Disability.* London: The Women's Press.

Morris, J. (1998a) *'Still Missing?', Volume 1: Disabled Children and the Children Act.* London: Who Cares? Trust.

Morris, J. (1998b) *Don't Leave us Out! Involving Disabled Children and Young People with Communication Impairments.* York: Joseph Rowntree Foundation.

Morris, J. (1999) *Foundations: Supporting Disabled Children and their Families, (N79) November.* York: Joseph Rowntree Foundation.

Morris, J. (2001) *That Kind of Life.* London: Scope.

Morrow, V. (1998) *Understanding Families: Children's Perspectives.* London: National Children's Bureau/Joseph Rowntree Foundation.

Mostert, M.P. (2001) 'Facilitated communication since 1995: A review of published studies.' *Journal of Autism and Developmental Disorders 31,* 3, pp.287–313.

Mukherjee, S., Beresford, B. and Sloper, P. (1999) *Unlocking Key Working: An Analysis and Evaluation of Key Worker Services for Families with Disabled Children.* Bristol: The Policy Press/Community Care.

Murray, P. (2000) 'Disabled children, parents and professionals: partnership on whose terms?' *Disability and Society 15,* 4, 683–698.

Murray, P. and Penman, J. (Eds) (1996) *Let Our Children Be – A Collection of Stories.* Sheffield: Parents With Attitude.

NCH Action for Children (1995) *All in the Family: Siblings and Disability.* London: NCH.

Noyes, J. (1999) *Voices and Choices: Young People who use Assisted Ventilation: Their Health and Social Care and Education.* London: HMSO.

Oliver, M. (1990) *The Politics of Disablement.* London: Macmillan.

Oliver, M. (1992) 'Changing the social relations of research production.' *Disability, Handicap and Society 7*, 101–114.

Oliver, M. (1993) 'Redefining disability: A challenge to research.' In J. Swain, V. Finkelstein, S. French, and M. Oliver (eds) *Disabling Barriers – Enabling Environments.* London: Sage.

Oliver, M. (1996) 'Defining impairment and disability: Issues at stake.' In C. Barnes and G. Mercer (eds) *Exploring the Divide: Illness and Disability.* Leeds: The Disability Press.

OPCS Surveys of Disability in Great Britain Report 6 (1989). London: HMSO.

Oswin, M. (1998) 'An historical perspective.' In C. Robinson and K. Stalker (eds) *Growing Up With Disability.* London: Jessica Kingsley Publishers.

People First Scotland (1996) *Special Schools... 'and now We are Different'.* Edinburgh: People First Scotland.

Potter, C. and Whittaker, C. (2001) *Enabling Communication in Children with Autism.* London: Jessica Kingsley Publishers.

Price, J. and Shildrick, M. (1998) 'Uncertain thoughts on the disabled body.' In M. Shildrick and J. Price (eds) *Vital Signs: Feminist Reconstructions of the Biological Body.* Edinburgh: Edinburgh University Press.

Priestley, M. (1998) 'Childhood disability and disabled childhoods: agendas for research.' *Childhood 5*, 2, 207–223.

Riddell, S. (2002) 'In 2001, the SEN and Disability Act became law.' *Children in Scotland,* January, 18–19.

Robinson, C. (1996) 'Breaks for disabled children.' In K. Stalker (ed) *Developments in Short-Term Care: Breaks and Opportunities.* London: Jessica Kingsley Publishers.

Robinson, C. and Stalker, K. (1998) *Growing Up with Disability.* Research Highlights in Social Work Series. London: Jessica Kingsley Publishers.

Rose, H. (1997) *Tom – A Gift in Disguise.* Findhorn: The Findhorn Press.

Russell, P. (1996a) 'Listening to children with special educational needs.' In R. Davie and D. Galloway (eds) *Listening to Children in Education.* London: David Fulton Publishers.

Russell, P. (1996b) 'Short term care: Parental perspectives.' In K. Stalker (ed) *Developments in Short Term Care: Breaks and Opportunities.* London: Jessica Kingsley Publishers.

Scottish Executive (2000) *The Same as You? A Review of Services for People with Learning Disabilities.* Edinburgh: The Scottish Executive.

Scottish Executive (2001) *For Scotland's Children.* Edinburgh: HMSO. Also available at: http://www.scotland.gov.uk/library3/education/fcsr07.asp

Scottish Office (1997) *Scotland's Children: The Children (Scotland) Act 1995 Regulations and Guidance, Vol. 1, Support and Protection for Children and their Families.* Edinburgh: HMSO.

Shakespeare, T. and Watson, N. (1997) 'Defending the social model.' In L. Barton and M. Oliver (eds) *Disability Studies: Past, Present and Future.* Leeds: The Disability Press.

Shakespeare, T. and Watson, N. (1998) 'Theoretical perspectives on research with disabled children.' In C. Robinson and K. Stalker (eds) *Growing Up With Disability.* Research Highlights in Social Work Series. London: Jessica Kingsley Publishers.

Shaw, L. (1998) 'Children's experiences of school.' In C. Robinson and K. Stalker (eds) *Growing Up with Disability.* London: Jessica Kingsley Publishers.

Shearer, A. (1980) *Handicapped Children in Residential Care: A Study of Policy Failure.* London: King's Fund Centre.

Shelley, P. (1998) 'Brothers and sisters are special too!' *Talking Sense,* Spring, 20–21.

Skar, L. and Tamm, M. (2001) 'My Assistant and I: Disabled children's and adolescents' roles and relationships to their assistants.' *Disability and Society 16,* 7, 917–931.

Smith, L.A. and Williams. J. M. (2001) 'Children's understandings of the physical, cognitive and social consequences of impairments.' *Child: Care, Health and Development 27,* 6, 603–617.

Social Services Inspectorate (1998) *Removing Barriers for Disabled Children: Inspection of Services to Disabled Children and their Families.* London: Department of Health.

Special Educational Needs & Disability Act (SENDA) (2001). Norwich: HMSO.

Stainton, T. and Besser, H. (1998) 'The positive impact of children with an intellectual disability on the family.' *Journal of Intellectual and Developmental Disability 23,* 1, 57–70.

Stalker, K. and Connors, C. (2003) 'Communicating with disabled children.' *Adoption and Fostering 27,* 1 (in press).

Stalker, K. and Reddish, S. (1995) *Supporting Disabled People in Scotland: An Overview of Health and Social Services.* Edinburgh: The Scottish Office.

Standards in Scotland's Schools Etc. Act (2000). Norwich: HMSO.

Stone, E. (2001) *Consulting with Disabled Children and Young People.* Findings 741. York: Joseph Rowntree Foundation.

Thomas, C. (1998) 'Parents and family: disabled women's stories about their childhood experiences.' In C. Robinson and K. Stalker (eds) *Growing Up with Disability.* London: Jessica Kingsley Publishers.

Thomas, C. (1999) *Female Forms: Experiencing and Understanding Disability.* Buckingham: Open University Press.

Thomson, G., Ward, K. and Wishart, J. (1995) 'The transition to adulthood for children with Down's Syndrome.' *Disability and Society 10*, 3, 325–340.

Tozer, R. (1996) 'My brother's keeper? Sustaining sibling support.' *Health and Social Care in the Community 4*, 3, 177–181.

United Nations (1989) *The Convention on the Rights of the Child.* Geneva: United Nations Children's Fund.

Waksler, F. (ed) (1991) *Studying the Social Worlds of Children: Sociological Readings.* London: Falmer.

Ward, L. (1997) *Seen and Heard: Involving Disabled Children and Young People in Research and Development Projects.* York: Joseph Rowntree Foundation.

Ward, L. (1999) 'Supporting disabled children and their families.' *Children and Society 13*, 394–400.

Ward, L. and Flynn, M. (1994) 'What matters most.' In M.H. Rioux and M. Bach (eds) *Disability is not Measles: New Research Paradigms in Disability.* Ontario: Roeher Institute.

Waters, J. (1996) 'Questionnaire to brothers and sisters of people with PWS.' *Prader-Willi Syndrome Association News*, December, 8–10.

Watson, N., Shakespeare, T., Cunningham-Burley, S., Barnes, C., Corker, M., Davis, J. and Priestley, M. (2000) *Life as a Disabled Child: A Qualitative Study of Young People's Experiences and Perspectives: Final Report to the ESRC Research Programme Children 5–16: 'Growing into the Twenty-First Century'.* www.esrc.ac.uk/curprog.html

Wheeler, S. (1993) 'A little brother; a lot of guilt.' *LINK 148*, Oct/Nov, 24–28.

Widdows, J. (1997) *A Special Needs for Inclusion: Children with Disabilities, Their Families and Everyday Life.* London: The Children's Society.

Williamson, H. and Butler, I. (1995) 'No-one ever listens to us: Interviewing children and young people.' In C. C. Luke and M. Davies (eds) *Participation and Empowerment in Child Protection.* London: Pitman.

Zarb, G. (1992) 'On the road to Damascus: First steps towards changing to relations of disability research production.' *Disability, Handicap and Society 7*, 125–138.

Information/Agreement Form
for Disabled Children Aged 8–10

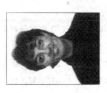

Dear......

My name is..............

I work at Stirling University.

This leaflet is about an exciting new project. In this project, I will be talking to children who use wheelchairs, who are blind, have epilepsy (fits) or some other condition. I want to find out about

- your favourite things to do
- your family and friends
- what you think about school
- what you want to do when you grow up

We hope the project will help us to help other disabled children.

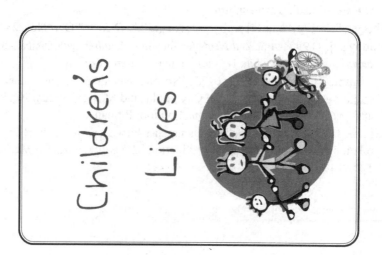

Children's Lives

Please read the Agreement Form in this leaflet or ask someone to read it to you.

If you would like me to come and see you, please write your name at the foot of the form. Or you can just make a cross, and ask someone to sign it for you.

If you don't want to be in the project, that's fine as well. You don't have to!

Bye for now

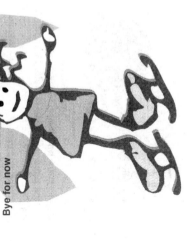

Do you want to be in this project?
If you do, I will come and see you at home 3 or 4 times.

We will have a chat about your life and things that matter to you.

If you like, you can do some drawings, record tapes and other activities. It could be fun!

You can ask me questions about the project anytime. I won't tell your parents or teachers what you said, unless you ask me to.

Don't worry if you need help speaking - we will talk whichever way suits you best.

When the project is over, I will send you a little book to keep, telling you what I have found out.

If you want to ask any questions now, you can phone me on 01786 - 467728 or send a fax: 01786 466319.

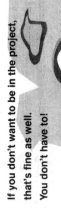

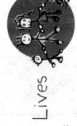

Children's Lives

AGREEMENT FORM:

- I have read the leaflet.

  OR

- the leaflet has been read to me
- I would like to take part in the project
- I know I can leave the project at any time if I change my mind.

NAME..

or NAME..

Signed on behalf of (child's name)....................

Please send this sheet back to me in the envelope provided. It doesn't need a stamp.

Information / Agreement Form for Disabled Children Aged 11–14

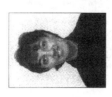

Dear.....

My name is.............
I work at Stirling University.

This leaflet is about an exciting new project. In this project, I will be talking to children who use wheelchairs, who are blind, have epilepsy (fits) or some other condition. I want to find out about

- your favourite things to do
- your family and friends
- what you think about school
- what you want to do when you grow up

We hope the project will help us to help other disabled children.

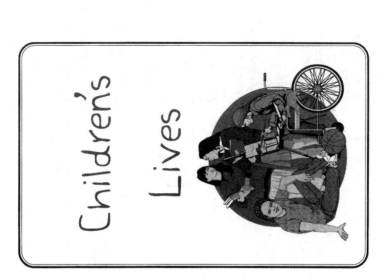

Children's Lives

Please read the Agreement Form in this leaflet. If you would like to be involved in the project, please write your name at the foot of the form. If it is hard for you to write, ask someone to sign it for you.

If you don't want to be in the project, that's fine as well.

You don't have to!

Bye for now

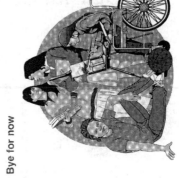

If you would like to take part, I will come and visit you at home 3 or 4 times.

The first time will be a chance for you to ask any questions about the project.

But you can ask me questions any time!

If you like, you can record tapes about yourself, or write a poem or a story.

Or if you prefer - we can just talk! I won't tell your parents or teachers what you said, unless you ask me to.

Don't worry if you need help speaking - we will communicate whichever way suits you best.

When the project is over, I will send you a book to keep, telling you what I have found out.

If you want to ask any questions now, you can phone me on 01786-467728 or send a fax: 01786 466319.

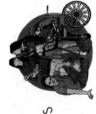

Children's Lives

AGREEMENT FORM:

- I have read the leaflet.

OR

- the leaflet has been read to me
- I would like to take part in the project
- I know I can leave the project at any time if I change my mind.

NAME..

or NAME..

Signed on behalf of (child's name)..........................

Please send this sheet back to me in the envelope provided. It doesn't need a stamp.

Information/Agreement Form for Siblings Aged 8–10

Dear.....

My name is.............
I work at Stirling University.

This leaflet is about an exciting new project. In this project, I will be talking to children who use wheelchairs, who are blind, have epilepsy (fits) or some other condition. I hope I can talk to their brothers and sisters as well. I want to find out:

- what you do together
- how you get on together
- any help you give your brother or sister
- any help you would like to have

We hope the project will help us to help other families.

Children's Lives

Please read the Agreement Form in this leaflet or ask someone to read it to you.

If you would like me to come and see you, please write your name at the foot of the form.

If you don't want to be in the project, that's fine as well. You don't have to - even if the rest of your family is in it.

Bye for now

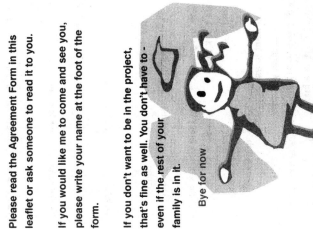

Do you want to be in this project? If your family takes part, I will come to your home 3 or 4 times.

If you like, you can do some drawings, record tapes and other activities. It could be fun!

You can ask me questions about the project anytime. I won't tell your parents what you said, unless you ask me to.

When the project is over, I will send you a little book to keep, telling you what I have found out.

If you want to ask any questions now, you can phone me on 01786 - 467728 or send a fax: 01786 466319.

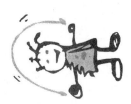

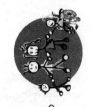

Children's Lives

AGREEMENT FORM:

- I have read the leaflet.

OR

- the leaflet has been read to me
- I would like to take part in the project
- I know I can leave the project at any time if I change my mind.

NAME...

or NAME...

Signed on behalf of (child's name)..................................

Please send this sheet back to me in the envelope provided. It doesn't need a stamp.

Information/Aggreement Form for Siblings Aged 11–14

Dear......

My name is..........
I work at Stirling University.

This leaflet is about a new research project. In this project, I will be talking to children who use wheelchairs, who are blind, have epilepsy (fits) or some other condition. I would also like to talk to their brothers and sisters. I want to hear your views about

- how you get on together
- whether people have explained your brother or sister's condition to you
- whether you are involved in family decisions
- whether you would like any information or support

We hope the results of the research will help us to help other other families with disabled children.

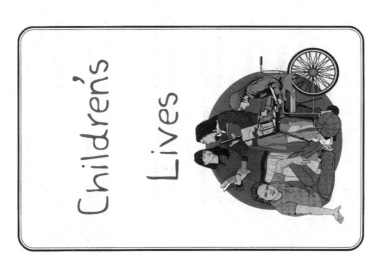

Children's Lives

Please read the Agreement Form in this leaflet. If you would like to be involved in the project, please write your name at the foot of the form.

If you don't want to be in the project, that's fine as well. You don't have to - even if other people in your family decide to go ahead.

Bye for now

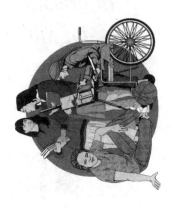

If your family decides to take part, I will come to your home 3 or 4 times.

The first time will be a chance for you to ask any questions about the project.

But you can ask me questions any time!

If you like, you can record tapes about yourself, or write a poem or a story.

Or if you prefer - we can just talk! I won't tell your parents what you said, unless you ask me to.

When the project is over, I will send you a book to keep, telling you what I have found out.

If you want to ask any questions now, you can phone me on 01786-467728 or send a fax: 01786 466319.

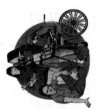

Children's Lives

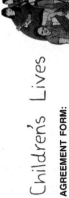

AGREEMENT FORM:

- I have read the leaflet.

OR

- the leaflet has been read to me
- I would like to take part in the project
- I know I can leave the project at any time if I change my mind.

NAME...

or NAME...

Signed on behalf of (child's name)....................

Please send this sheet back to me in the envelope provided. It doesn't need a stamp.

Guide for Second Visit to Disabled Children aged 8–10 and those with Learning Difficulties

Remember to take: all the graphic and printed material plus drawing paper and felt-tips!

Remind child about what was discussed at first meeting, especially how s/he can stop the interview if s/he wants. Remind her/him there are no right answers: we're just interested to hear about her/his life and what s/he thinks about things. Remind her/him about confidentiality.

1. Begin by looking at pictures/photos or listening to tape and asking child about them.

For example, ask her/him to explain what the picture is about, why s/he chose to draw that, etc. This discussion could last 5–10 minutes as a warm-up but is also a chance for the child to identify aspects of life which are important to her/him. It is what child says about drawing/photos etc. which count as data, not the items themselves (which if lent to researcher should be returned to child). Be positive about the picture/tape and thank child for doing it.

Play back some of the tape to child if s/he wants to hear it or let her/him play it back and be in charge of the tape.

2. Who are the important people in your life?

Give child a spidergram (see Appendix G) and ask her/him to fill in 'Who is important to me?' Ask her/him to fill in names of the most important people in red and others who are quite important in green (if child can't write/see, then researcher asks questions and fills in). Stress that s/he doesn't need to fill in all the boxes and that s/he can make more boxes or add more names if s/he likes. Ask child to talk about each person:

- who are they and how do you know them? (if not obvious)
- where do they live?
- what sort of things do you do together?
- why are they important/why do you like X?

3.   Ask child to describe a typical day, (i) at school and (ii) at the weekend.

Can you tell me what you do on an ordinary day? Say like yesterday – when did you get up? What did you have for breakfast? How did you get to school? Repeat similar question for a weekend day.

Adapt according to child's ability. Ask supplementary questions as necessary as child recounts day, e.g. who else was there? What was that like? What was the best thing that happened yesterday? What was the worst thing?

4.   What are the favourite things you like doing, not just yesterday, but any day?

Why do you like doing that?

Use pictures as prompts if necessary, but not before child has given own responses where these are forthcoming. If it seems appropriate, ask child if s/he wants to draw her/his favourite activity.

5.   Are there any things you really don't like doing?

What things? What don't you like about them?

6.   Are there some things you are quite good at?

What are they? What do you like about them?

7.   Are there any things you find difficult to do?

What are they? Why are they difficult?

8.   At school

I'd like to hear more about your school. What do you think about school?
If not already covered:

What do you do there? (prompt: what did you do there today?)

What's your teacher like?

What do you do in the playground?

Have you got any special friends?

What's the best thing about school?

What's the worst thing?

Have you ever been bullied at school?

(if so) What happened?

Have you talked to anyone about it?

9. Word Choice.

Give child Word Choice sheet (see Appendix I) and felt-tip: ask her/him to circle all the words that fit her/him at school:

happy	fed-up	friendly
lazy	helpful	sad
dreamy	jokey	sporty
keen	naughty	brainy

Ask why the child has circled each word. Validate positive feelings. Where a more negative feeling is identified, ask if it's okay to feel like that, or if s/he would like things to be different.

10. Are there any things you need help to do (because of...)?

Prompt if necessary. If so:

What things?

Who gives you help?

Is s/he good at helping you?

If you were giving her/him a score out of 10 for the way s/he helps you, what score would you give her/him?

Why?

11. Good/bad things: lifeline

Give child lifeline (see Appendix H) on a big piece of paper and explain how it works. Ask her/him to fill in events/people that make life good or bad wherever s/he wants along the line.

Life very good	good	life okay	bad	Life very bad

Ask child about each thing s/he has filled in: what is it about? What makes it good/bad? Do other people know this is something s/he likes/dislikes? What would make it better?

12. Brothers and sisters

Give child illustrated cards to complete (see Appendix L).

Sisters:	**Brothers:**
Name	Name
Age	Age
Best things about her	Best things about him
Worst things	Worst things
We have fun when	We have fun when
She annoys me when	He annoys me when
I annoy her when	I annoy him when
We get on together	We get on together

Ask child to say a bit more about her/his answers as appropriate.

13. **Ask child if s/he would like to do another drawing or record some more on tape for next time. If child isn't keen, just leave it.**

Guide for Third Visit to Disabled Children aged 8–10 and those with Learning Difficulties

Begin by checking child is happy to go ahead and talk. Remind her/him about confidentiality and the way in which s/he can stop the interview at any time.

1. **If child has drawn a picture or taped something, begin by looking at/listening to that and talking about it.**

2. **Ask child what has been happening since you last met/what s/he has been doing.**

3. **Ask what s/he would like to talk about today/if there is anything special s/he would like to talk about.**

4. **Choices Chart**

I'd like to know how much you make choices about your life and how much other people help you decide or maybe choose things for you. Can you have a look at this chart and tick the boxes which show who decides things. If you like, you can do a big tick for the people that decide most often and a little tick for the people who sometimes decide. So if your mum usually decides what time you get up, maybe during school terms, but you decide at the weekends, you give your mum a big tick and give 'me' a little tick.

	me	mum	dad	brother	sister	someone else (who?)

What time I get up

What I wear

What I do after school

What I do at weekends

What I have for tea

What I do on my birthday

Who I play with

Do you think you have enough say about things in your life?

5. Map of where I live

Show child the map-making materials. Explain how s/he can make up a map of the area where s/he lives and any places s/he knows about or goes to round about her/his house.

As s/he is doing it or when s/he has finished, ask the child to tell you about the different places, and about her/his visits to them, what s/he does there, etc.

Ask if there are any places s/he hasn't been to or can't go to and why. Ask child if s/he knows other children living round about and if s/he plays with them.

6. Sentence completion

Ask child to complete these sentences:

My favourite TV programme is…

My most valuable possession is…

I feel happy when…

I feel sad when…

When I grow up I would like to…

Something I am really good at is…

Something I find difficult is…

After the child has done all these, ask her/him to say more about any that seem of particular relevance, e.g. why is something difficult/what would help make it better?

7. **If you had a magic wand and you could wish for something to happen, what would you wish?**

    Why would you wish that?

    Is there anything else you would wish for, if you could have another wish?

    If so, what would it be?

    What about your disability? Would you change anything about that?

8. **If I asked you how much of the time you feel happy, would you say:**

    - most of the time

    - some of the time

    - not much of the time?

    Why is that?

(*If appropriate*) What would help make you feel happy more of the time?

9. **Services and professionals**

NB: if possible, before this visit ask the parents about the services/professionals with whom the child has contact, and what the child calls each person.

Sometimes children get help from people outside the family. When you go to school, the teachers help you to learn things. If you're not feeling well, you might go to the doctor and s/he will try to make you feel better. The next questions are about some of the people you might have seen who would try to help you in different ways.

Give child, one by one, cards with pictures of services/professionals and ask some of the following questions, as appropriate:

    - have you ever met a social worker?

If necessary, prompt child: 'Your mum told me that Ann comes to see you.'

    - do you know why s/he comes to see you?

    - what does s/he talk to you about?

- if you were going to give her/him a mark out of 10 for how helpful s/he is, what mark would you give her/him?
- why have you given her/him that mark?

or (for a buildings based service):

- have you ever been to a hospital?
- what happened there?
- why did you go there?
- what was it like in hospital?

Cards will be of:

teacher

social worker (*explain if necessary*)

doctor

hospital

respite care unit/link family

playscheme/club

- is there anyone else that comes to see you?
- is there anywhere else you go?
- do you know anywhere else that helps children?

10. A problem/worry – spidergram

A lot of people worry about different things. Do you ever worry about anything?
If so, ask her/him to do a spidergram: the problem can be written in the body of the spider, the top four legs 'What causes the problem?' and the bottom four, 'How does it make you feel?'
Do you ever worry about your disability?

11. The future

Pretend you are grown up, as old as your mum and dad – what do you want to be doing when you are that age?

Where would you like to live? What sort of house? Who would you like to live with?

Would you like to have a job? If so, what sort of job? What about your disability?

Will you need any help to do the things you want when you're grown up?

What sort of help?

12: Is there anything else you would like to talk about?

Thank child for talking to you and for the drawings / tapes. Explain that when you have finished the project s/he will get a little book about what s/he and all the other children have said.

A Spidergram

People in my Life

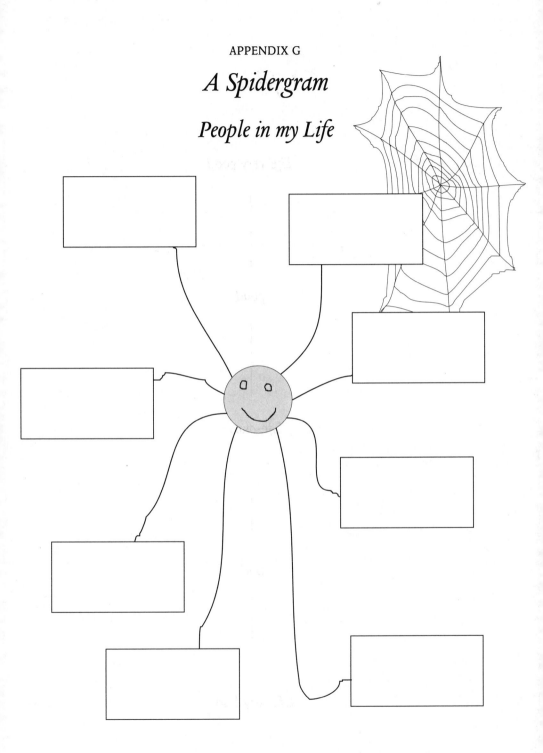

Lifeline

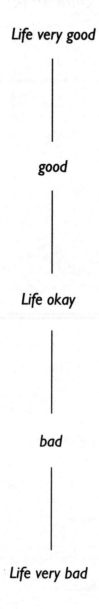

Life very good

good

Life okay

bad

Life very bad

Word Choice Sheet

Me at School

friendly	sad	sporty	bored
fed-up	helpful	jokey	naughty
happy	lazy	dreamy	keen

Interview Guide for Siblings aged 8–10

Introduction

At the start, remind children what was discussed at first meeting, especially that they can 'pass' on a question or stop the interview if they want. Remind them there are no right answers: their views are important and that's what we want to hear. Also remind them about confidentiality.

Start by looking at/listening to any tape, story or poem the children have prepared and discuss that for a while, e.g. ask them to explain what the poem is about, why they chose to write about that, etc. This discussion could last about 5–10 minutes as a warm-up, but is also a chance for the child to identify aspects of life that are important to her/him, as well as any more specifically relating to their disabled brother/sister. It is what kids say about the material that counts as data, not the material itself (which if lent to the researcher should be returned to the child). Be positive about the poem/tape and thank young people for doing them.

Ask kids to describe a typical day: (i) at school, (ii) at the weekend. Can you tell me what you do on an ordinary day? Say like yesterday – when did you get up? What did you have for breakfast? How did you get to school?

Repeat similar question for a weekend day.

Ask them if they would like to draw a picture of their brother or sister (if they haven't already done so) and to talk about it.

Spending time together

Do you spend much time with X?

What sort of things do you do together?

Do you ever help look after X?

If so, how do you help?

Do you ever help X do things that might be difficult for her to do?

If I said to you, 'I hear you've got a sister called X but I've never met her. What's she like?' what would you say to me?

Word choice

How do you (each) and X get on together?

Do you have fun together?

(If so) what sort of funny things do you do together?

Lots of brothers and sisters have times when they don't get on so well. Do you ever have arguments or fight?

(If so) what do you fight about?

X's disability

X can't walk/can't see very well/finds it hard to learn some things. Has anyone ever talked to you about that? (If so, who? What did they say?)

Have your mum and dad ever talked to you about X's (disability)?

Do you ever think you would like to know more about her (disability)?

If so, is there someone you could ask about that?

Do you ever worry about X? Or anything to do with her (disability)?

What do you worry about?

Have you talked to anyone about that?

What's it like having X as a sister (good things/not so good things)?

Spidergram

Can you write in the boxes some words that say how you feel about X?

Do you think having X for a sister is any different from having a sister without a disability?

If so, in what way?

Does having X around ever limit what you can do?

Do you have any friends, or do you know other children, who have a brother or sister with a disability?

If so, do you talk to them about it?

Do your friends know X?

How do they get on with her?

Support for siblings

Some families with disabled children have a social worker coming to see them.

Has a social worker ever been to see you?

(If so) do you know why she came to see you?

Did she help you in any way?

Some places have groups for children/young people with disabled brothers or sisters, where they can get together and talk about things. Have you ever been in a group like that?

If so, what was it like?

If not, would you like to go along to a group like that, if there was one near here?

Do you ever feel you would like to talk to someone outside the family about X?

The future

What do you think X will be doing in 20 years' time?

What do you think you will be doing in 20 years' time?

Will you be doing things together then?

(If so) what sort of things?

Thank you for answering all these questions. Is there anything you want to tell me?

Is there anything you'd like to ask me?

Word Choice Sheet

My Brother

different	clever	funny
sad	happy	hyper
lazy	annoying	cool
helpful	odd	naughty
kind	sleepy	embarassing
loving	moody	stubborn

Children's Lives

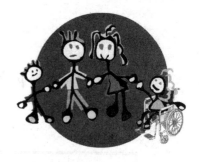

Sisters

Name ....

Age ....

Best things about her ....

Worst things about her ....

We have fun when ....

She annoys me when ....

I annoy her when ....

We get on together ....

Subject Index

Author Index